AHCC

The Medical Breakthrough in Natural Immunotherapy

FRED PESCATORE, MD

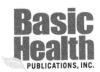

Basic Health
PUBLICATIONS, INC.

The information contained in this book is based upon the research and personal and professional experiences of the authors. It is not intended as a substitute for consulting with your physician or other healthcare provider. Any attempt to diagnose and treat an illness should be done under the direction of a healthcare professional.

The publisher does not advocate the use of any particular healthcare protocol but believes the information in this book should be available to the public. The publisher and authors are not responsible for any adverse effects or consequences resulting from the use of the suggestions, preparations, or procedures discussed in this book. Should the reader have any questions concerning the appropriateness of any procedures or preparation mentioned, the authors and the publisher strongly suggest consulting a professional healthcare advisor.

Basic Health Publications, Inc.
An imprint of Turner Publishing Company
Nashville, TN 37209
www.turnerbookstore.com

Library of Congress Cataloging-in-Publication Data

Pescatore, Fred
    AHCC : the medical breakthrough in natural immunotherapy /
Fred Pescatore.
        p. cm.
    ISBN 978-1-59120-280-6 (pbk) | ISBN 978-1-68162-693-2 (hc)
    1. Biological response modifiers. 2. Cancer—Alternative treatment.
3. Mushrooms—Therapeutic use. 4. Glucans—Therapeutic use. I. Title.

    RC271.B53P47   2010
    616.99'4061—dc22

                                                    2009045283

Manuscript and research consultant: Dan Kenner, PhD
Editor: Diana Drew
Typesetting/Book design: Gary A. Rosenberg
Cover design: Mike Stromberg

Printed in the United States of America

10   9   8   7   6   5   4   3   2

Contents

*With special gratitude to Dr. Yasuo Komiyama,
Professor Emeritus of Kansai Medical University in Japan,
an author and dedicated researcher in the field of AHCC,
for providing background materials that made
the publication of this book possible.*

Introducing AHCC, a Food Supplement from Japan with Medical Applications

AHCC®—one of the world's best-researched natural products—is a unique extract of cultured mycelia (roots) of Japanese medicinal mushrooms. It is used in over a thousand clinics and hospitals worldwide, mainly as an adjuvant to cancer treatment. AHCC is used in this medical context without hesitation by doctors because it is as well researched as any conventional prescription drug. The quality control of AHCC is so stringent that it would easily qualify as a licensed pharmaceutical, but the manufacturers believe that this would limit its availability to the many people in Japan—healthy people, who use it as a preventive as well as for a variety of other purposes. Because it is actually a food, even though it is often put into capsules, it is extremely safe for anyone to take, including children, pets, frail elderly people, and patients who have undergone surgery. AHCC is a mushroom-based food supplement with properties that are clearly different from other mushroom-based health foods available on the market. More than two decades have passed since the development of AHCC and its appearance in the marketplace. This book explores AHCC in depth and explains how it is used in clinics in Japan and other parts of the world, probes its safety, delves into how it is manufactured, and examines the scientific evidence supporting its

striking versatility and profound effectiveness for a wide variety
of conditions.

It is vital for each of us to understand our body and its
condition of health or disease in order to make appropriate
decisions about health care. Treatment using only conventional drugs, with their inevitable deleterious side effects, raises the
question of whether decisions about treatment should be made
by the medical practitioner or the patient. Patients often ask
whether there are any alternative or complementary treatments
available for a medical condition affecting them. AHCC, because
of its safety, efficacy, and the body of scientific evidence supporting its use, appears to be a safe choice for almost anyone for the
treatment and prevention of a wide range of health conditions.
This book will introduce you to AHCC and expand your knowledge of one of the most important food supplements available
on the market today.

CHAPTER 1

What Is AHCC?

AHCC®, a novel nutraceutical sold under a registered trademark of Amino Up Chemical Co. Ltd., is a mushroom-based functional food developed through joint research by Professor Toshihiko Okamoto in the Department of Pharmacology, Tokyo University, and Amino Up Chemical Co. Ltd. It was developed as a food product that could be used as a therapeutic aid for lifestyle-related diseases, including liver diseases and diabetes, in particular, and its creators had high expectations for its use in supporting immunity in cancer patients. The high expectations of the developers of this product have been fulfilled beyond their greatest hopes.

AHCC AS A HEALTH FOOD

In Japan, health foods—also called *functional foods, dietary supplements,* and *supplements*—fall under the category of *foods* but these names do not reflect the beneficial nature of these products. AHCC can be said to have achieved the pharmacological and medical reliability of a pharmaceutical product, based on the profusion of research on its pharmacological action as well as the controlled clinical trials and informal studies carried out in cooperation with numerous doctors, clinics, hospitals, and universities. It could be called an *immunostimulating food,* which would be a unique category of functional food. It strengthens the immune system, and therefore bolsters the physiology of the whole body.

AHCC: A HEALTH FOOD THAT HAS THE SAME LEVEL OF QUALITY CONTROL AS PHARMACEUTICAL DRUGS

Even though AHCC is classified as a health food, it is used by medical experts and patients as a functional food, a food specifically aimed at influencing physiological function. Amino Up Chemical Co. Ltd. in Sapporo, Japan, the original manufacturer of AHCC, uses manufacturing and quality-control methods equivalent to those used in making pharmaceutical products in accordance with the GMP (Good Manufacturing Practice) guidelines for the standards of manufacture and quality control of drugs.

GMP guidelines require the following:

1. Human error should be at a minimum.

2. Contamination of the drug and changes in quality of the drug should be prevented.

3. The factory should be designed to ensure high quality and aim at improving the quality of the drug by setting strict standards related to the manufacture and storage of the drug and the structural layout of the facility. In addition, complaint handling, complaint reports, and record maintenance related to the drug are mandatory.

AHCC also adheres to international quality and safety standards, including the HACCP9000 system. This system is a combination of HACCP (Hazard Analysis Critical Control Point) systems, which is an international-level hygiene-control system for foods and ISO9002 (International Organization for Standardization 9002), which is a quality-assurance system, thus ensuring complete quality assurance. To prove that its quality conforms to these requirements, the company has to allow inspections by a third-party organization. When the company passes these inspections, its methodology gets the HACCP certification, ISO certification, and Japanese nutritional supplement GMP accreditation (see Table 1.1).

TABLE 1.1 HACCP, ISO, AND GMP CERTIFICATIONS

HACCP (Hazard Analysis Critical Control Point)
A scientific control system based on the prevention of hazards.

ISO (International Organization for Standardization)
A set of international standards of quality to strengthen the trust of distributors and consumers by establishing a stringent quality-assurance system.

GMP (Good Manufacturing Practice)
These are the standards related to product control and quality control of a drug. GMP sets the standards for both structural setup and procedural control to ensure high quality by preventing poor handling and contamination. GMP requires rigorous methods of control of the manufacturing process.

In the manufacturing and quality assurance of AHCC, the manufacturers have conformed to the level of manufacturing and quality assurance on a par with international manufacturing and quality-assurance standards of pharmaceutical drugs.

AHCC: A LIQUID CULTURE OF BASIDIOMYCETES, EXTRACTED AND REFINED BY A PROPRIETARY METHOD

The common name for a large fungus is *mushroom*. Mushrooms are in the family of true fungi, but true fungi also include molds; mushrooms are scientifically referred to as basidiomycetes (see Figure 1.1). Shiitake, matsutake, maitake, nameko, and agaricus (the common field mushroom) mushrooms that are used as food are typical basidiomycetes. Mushrooms are believed to have had a therapeutic effect on disease since ancient times. In

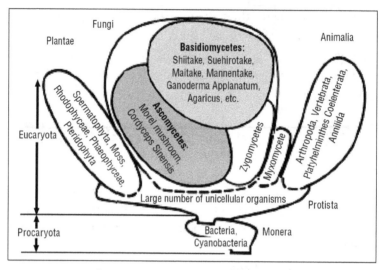

Figure 1.1 Classification of mushrooms

Chinese medicine, certain mushrooms, such as the famous reishi, are considered to be effective in fighting cancer. The mushrooms used as food are just a part and not the entire mushroom. The mushrooms also have mycelia (the hairlike root structure), which absorb nutrients. The mycelium bores through the soil or attaches to wood; we usually don't use it as food (see Figure 1.2).

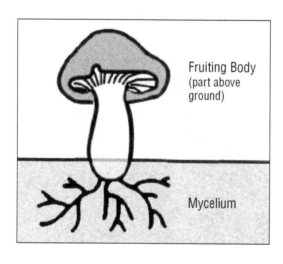

Fruiting Body
(part above
ground)

Mycelium

Figure 1.2
Fruiting body and
mycelium of the
mushroom

Although most mushroom-based products considered to be beneficial in combating disease are processed from the edible portion, the so-called "fruiting body," the concept in producing AHCC has been to focus on extraction from the mycelium culture, which is the source of production of the active ingredients of mushrooms.

Large-scale culture of these mycelia has been made possible in recent years and has been put to practical use in the AHCC production plants. Shiitake (*Lentinus edodes*) mushrooms are used as one of the raw materials of AHCC.

WHY A MUSHROOM PRODUCT?

Why not just eat the mushrooms whole? Mushrooms are composed of large molecules and have a spongy quality, so digestion is not always optimal. One significant component in healing mushrooms is β-glucan (beta glucan). This substance has a very large molecular size, so large that some scientists thought it might even be too large for the human body to absorb. Further breakdown by the culturing process makes the nutrients in mushrooms more absorbable and therefore more readily available to the body.

MANUFACTURING PROCESS OF AHCC

Figure 1.3 is a diagram of the manufacturing process of AHCC. AHCC is manufactured by culturing the mycelia of basidiomycetes (the mushroom root structure) for an extended period in a tank. Several types of mycelia are initially cultured to form a colony (a mass of mycelia) and then further cultured in a large tank for forty-five to sixty days. After the culture is completed, the product is subjected to enzyme reaction, sterilization, concentration, and freeze-drying. The culturing of basidiomycetes can extend up to a period of forty-five to sixty days in the man-

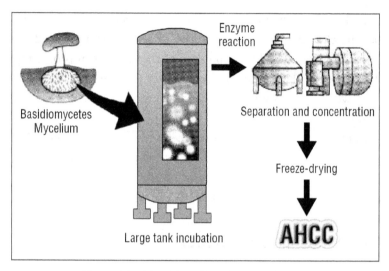

Figure 1.3   Manufacturing process of AHCC

ufacturing of AHCC. This long-term culturing has been made possible only by the development of a proprietary manufacturing method and culturing system (see Figure 1.4).

Because the fungi are extremely delicate, it is vital to maintain high air pressure and ensure the aseptic maintenance of equipment. These manufacturing methods prevent contamination from foreign microorganisms and facilitate a stable culturing environment for the necessary period of time—at least six weeks. Decay of the culture solution, due to contamination by microorganisms, is strictly prevented. Computer monitoring, to carefully control the culture conditions (temperature, stirring conditions, etc.), is essential when using such large tanks. There is probably no other similar product among health foods cultured for as long as AHCC.

Generally speaking, health foods of mushroom origin are natural products; hence the components may differ, depending on the producer and the manufacturing method. In the case of AHCC, however, the chemical constituents and the quality are consistently maintained. This is achieved through attention to every detail of the manufacturing process, using the latest technology. The consistent quality of AHCC can be said to be one of the factors that sets it apart from other health foods.

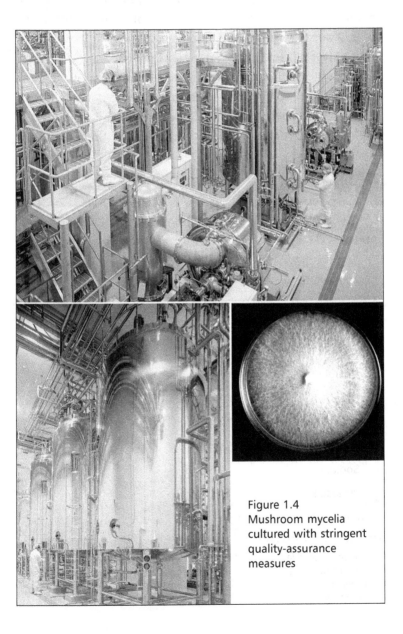

Figure 1.4
Mushroom mycelia
cultured with stringent
quality-assurance
measures

CHEMICAL COMPOSITION OF AHCC

Table 1.2 shows the components of AHCC granules. It is difficult to understand why AHCC has such a powerful effect on the immune system when we look at these components individually. It is noteworthy that carbohydrates make up almost 50 percent of AHCC. Most of these carbohydrates are polysaccharides. Besides the beta glucan (β-glucan, the principal ingredient of the most common mushroom-based health foods), these polysaccharides contain alpha glucans (α-glucans), which have a low molecular weight. The activity of AHCC is attributed to the presence of these α-glucans.

TABLE 1.2 COMPONENTS OF AHCC GRANULES	
Component	Componential analysis value (per 100g)
Description	Light brown granules; have a distinctive flavor and odor
Carbohydrates	44.0g
Fats	37.3g
Proteins	7.2g
Vitamin B_1	0.3g
Vitamin B_2	0.3g
Niacin	0.3g
Dietary fiber	5.7g
Minerals	4.5g
Sodium	550mg
Potassium	1,200mg
Water content	1.3g

Tested by Hokkaido Pharmaceutical Association's Public Health Inspection Center.

While monosaccharides are an efficient source of energy, polysaccharides are not direct nutrients, but play an important part in regulating various body functions. Recent research has shown that polysaccharides stimulate the immune system and therefore they can have a beneficial effect on a wide range of diseases.

WHAT ARE POLYSACCHARIDES?

Polysaccharides are relatively complex carbohydrates. Polysaccharides are the active elements in many health foods made from plants and mushrooms. Many manufacturers emphasize polysaccharide content, especially when it comes to health foods made from mushrooms.

Since AHCC is a mushroom-based health food, polysaccharides are important constituents. As the word implies, *polysaccharides* are formed by the bonding of "numerous monosaccharides." Glucose, a well-known sugar, also known as blood sugar, is a monosaccharide. Several of these monosaccharides are connected in a chain to form a polysaccharide. Examples of polysaccharides include oligosaccharides, starch, and cellulose. Dietary fibers, which help in regulating the gastrointestinal tract, also fall into the category of polysaccharides (see Figure 1.5).

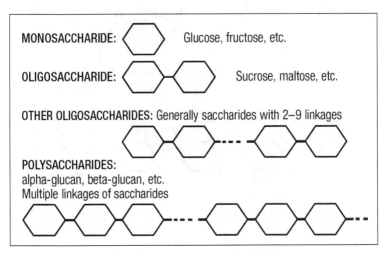

Figure 1.5 Polysaccharides

Polysaccharides are complex carbohydrates that are digested and absorbed more gradually than simple sugars. Monosaccharides, or simple sugars, can sometimes cause adverse effects because of their sudden impact on blood sugar regulation, but there is no reason to be concerned about adverse effects from the consumption of AHCC, in which polysaccharides are the principal components.

β-GLUCAN AND α-GLUCAN

Most of the polysaccharides in mushroom-based health foods are β-glucans. In very simple terms, *beta* refers to the types of linkages of glucose molecules; α-glucan has "alpha" bonds of glucose. As shown in Figure 1.6, the difference between a beta bond and an alpha bond is in the links between the molecules of glucose.

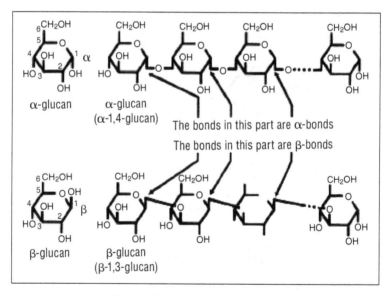

Figure 1.6 α-glucan and β-glucan

Our bodies do not contain enzymes to digest β-glucans, but we do secrete the digestive enzyme α-amylase, which digests α-glucans.

ACTIVE COMPONENTS OF AHCC

The polysaccharides that comprise the principal ingredients of AHCC include β-glucan and acetylated α-glucan. This acetylated α-glucan is the specific element that is unique to AHCC (see Figure 1.7). Glucans are polysaccharides and these polysaccharides are known to have various bioactive effects.

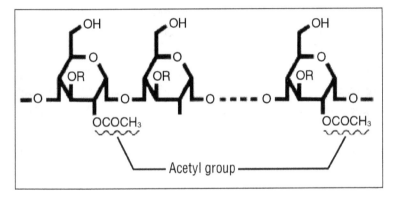

Figure 1.7 Active component of AHCC: Acetylated α-1,4 glucan

Acetylating means chemically adding an acetyl group (CH3CO–) to glucan. Although there is almost no acetylated α-glucan in the components of the mushroom itself, it is a constituent that is produced by culturing the mushroom.

This acetylated α-glucan has a comparatively low molecular weight (around 5,000 daltons). Normally, the molecular weight of β-glucan is in the range of tens to hundreds of thousands of daltons. This is believed to cause variable effects in the body because of individual differences in how it is digested. Although high molecular weight β-glucans are difficult to digest and absorb, they do demonstrate some immunopotentiating action by stimulating the intestinal tract. The acetylated α-glucans, however, demonstrate a direct systemic immunopotentiating action after they are digested and absorbed.

SAFETY OF AHCC

GLPs (Good Laboratory Practices—standards for clinical research protocols on the safety of medicines) were implemented in Japan in 1983 as the standard for animal tests. GLP provides standards for toxicity tests in animal testing. Apart from general toxicity tests, standards for special toxicity tests, such as reproduction/generation tests, carcinogenesis tests, dependence tests, and the like, have also been developed. In the toxicity tests, a quality-assurance unit must conduct the checks and all documents showing the procedures of the toxicity tests must be maintained to confirm that the tests are implemented according to the regulations. Inspections are carried out according to the regulations provided by the Japanese Health and Labor Ministry.

Safety studies have been conducted from the beginning of the development of AHCC, according to the GLP standards. Table 1.3 shows some of the results of safety tests carried out according to GLP standards. No toxicity was found with AHCC.

SCIENTIFIC RESEARCH CONDUCTED WORLDWIDE

AHCC was launched onto the market after confirming its safety through animal testing. After it was put on the market for direct sale, the use of AHCC was adopted by various medical institutions without any organized medical tests and without any compilation of clinical data. The AHCC Research Association, established in 1994, consists of professionals from medical institutions and universities, all working to prove AHCC's medical reliability. The association grows every year, and the 15th International AHCC Symposium, conducted in 2007, included approximately 350 participants, with more than 70 representing eight foreign countries. At this symposium, scientists presented reports on basic research, as well as research relating to clinical and safety issues.

TABLE 1.3 SAFETY TEST RESULTS OF AHCC ACCORDING TO GLP STANDARDS	
SINGLE ORAL ADMINISTRATION TOXICITY TEST	
Test animal	SD rats (5-week-old SPF male and 6-week-old female, 10 each)
Dose	12,500mg/kg weight (maximum dose)
Result	No death in either group
	LD50 > 12,500mg/kg by oral administration of AHCC
SINGLE INTRAPERITONEAL ADMINISTRATION TOXICITY TEST	
Test animal	SD rats (5-week-old SPF male and 6-week-old female, 5 each)
Dose	2,500mg/kg weight (maximum dose): total 6 groups of 10,500, 8,840, 7,430, 6,250mg/kg weight
Result	Toxic activity was not seen in intraperitoneal administration of AHCC.
	Male: LD50 = 8,490mg/kg, estimated fatal dose = 7,430mg/kg
	Female: LD50 = 9,849mg/kg and estimated fatal dose = 8,340mg/kg

At this symposium, discussions were held to further improve the reliability in AHCC research and the following issues concerning use of AHCC for patients were identified:

- First and foremost, AHCC is a food product.

- Research must be conducted with patient consent.

- Research protocols must be conducted under physician supervision and not interfere with normal medical treatment, nor be legally ambiguous with respect to liability, informed consent and third party payment coverage.

- The information obtained is to be strictly managed and maintained.

Almost all cases researched were with patients simultaneously undergoing medical treatment. The AHCC Research Association has compiled several thousand cases and examined the relationship between the intake of AHCC and immunity.

DEVELOPMENT OF AND RESEARCH INTO AHCC

So far, there have been volumes of research and test reports related to AHCC. The main points raised by this research are introduced in this book, but it may not be possible to give a complete overview of all of the research and development relating to AHCC. The inset "AHCC Research History" summarizes research into AHCC to date.

AHCC Research History

April 1986: AHCC development

September 1987: Basic research initiated by honorary Professor Okamoto Toshihiko of the College of Pharmacy, Tokyo University and Amino Up Chemical Co. Ltd.

April 1989: Joint research with the Hokkaido Industrial Research Institute and Hokkaido University Department of Agriculture: "Application in Physiologically Active Substances and Functional Foods That Use Basidiomycetes."

November 1992: Special Dietary Supplements Society, "Report on Activation of NK Cells in Cancer Patients with AHCC," UCLA Drew University, All-American Special Dietary Supplement Society's Academic Prize

August 1994: 10th International AIDS Conference (Yokohama), "Report on AHCC Immunotherapy in AIDS Patients," UCLA Drew University

October 1994: Founding of AHCC Research Association: Full-scale joint research started with regard to anticancer action of AHCC between domestic research institutes, including Hokkaido University Department of Medicine, Teikyo University Department of Pharmacy, and Kansai Medical School and Medical Institutes

May 1997: The 32nd European Surgical Society, "AHCC Immunotherapy for Liver Cancer Patients," Professors Soichiro Takai and Yasuo Kamiyama, Chief of Surgery, Kansai Medical University

May 1997: 4th Japan Cancer Prevention Society, "Anti-Mutagenic Activity of AHCC Which Is Extracted from Basidiomycetes Culture," Amino Up Chemical Co. Ltd.

August 1997: Amino Up Chemical Co. Ltd., "Preventive Effects of AHCC on Carbon Tetrachloride Induced Liver Injury in Mice," *Natural Medicine* 51, no. 4 (1997): 310–315

May 1998: Critical Appraisal of Unconventional/Alternative Interventions for Carcinoma of the Prostate: "Effects of AHCC (Active Hexose Correlated Compound) in Both the Prevention and Treatment of Carcinoma," B. Sun & K. Kosuna, Amino Up Chemical Co. Ltd.

May 1998: 33rd European Surgical Society, "Effects of AHCC in Prevention of Postoperative Relapse in Liver Cell Cancer Patients," Professors Soichiro Takai and Yasuo Kamiyama, Chief of Surgery, Kansai Medical School

July 1998: 5th Japan Cancer Prevention Society, "Macrophage Activation and Tumor Cell Proliferation Control Elements in Basidiomycetes Culture Extracts (AHCC)," Amino Up Chemical Co. Ltd.

September 1998: 57th Convention of the Japanese Cancer Association, "Search for AHCC (Basidiomycetes Culture Extract) Activators by the Macrophage Induction Function and Blood Cancer Cell Proliferation Control Action," Amino Up Chemical Co. Ltd.; and "Protection Effects of Active Hexose Correlated Compound (AHCC) in Cytosine Arabinoside-Induced Depilation Model," Amino Up Chemical Co. Ltd.

September 1998: Kazuhiro Matsushita, Hokkaido University, Cancer Research and Pathology, "Effect of Metastasis Control of Breast Cancer in Rats by Concomitant Use of AHCC and Anticancer Drug UFT," *Anticancer Drugs* 9 (1998): 343–350

October 1998: 34th Japan Liver Cancer Workshop, "Prognostic Effect of Administering AHCC as Postoperative Supplementary Treatment for Liver Cells Cancer," Youichi Matsui, Primary Surgery, Kansai Medical School

November 1998: Impact of Biotechnology on Cancer (NCE France), "Effect of Basidiomycetes Culture Extract AHCC on Reducing the Side Effects of Anticancer Drugs," Amino Up Chemical Co. Ltd.

March 1999: 119th Convention of the Pharmaceutical Society of Japan, "Effect of Active Hexose Correlated Compound (AHCC) on Streptozotocin-Induced Diabetic Rat," Amino Up Chemical Co. Ltd.; and "Effect of AHCC in Reducing the Hepatic Toxicity Caused by Anticancer Drugs," Amino Up Chemical Co. Ltd.

April 1999: 90th Convention of the American Association of Cancer Research, "Effect of AHCC in Reducing the Side Effects Caused by Anticancer Drugs," Amino Up Chemical Co. Ltd.

April 1999: 34th Convention of the European Surgical Society, "Effect of AHCC in Improving the Prognosis of Patients after Liver Surgery," Yasuo Kamiyama, Primary Surgery, Kansai Medical University

October 1999: Amino Up Chemical Co. Ltd., "Protective Effect of Active Hexose Correlated Compound (AHCC) on the Onset of Diabetes Induced by Streptozotocin in the Rat," *Biomedical Research* 20, no. 3 (1999): 145–152

May 2000: Katsuaki Uno, Comfort Hospital, "Effect of Plant-Derived Polysaccharide Extracts (AHCC) on Cancer Patients—Effect on Performance Status of Immunological Parameters," *Biotherapy* 14, no. 3 (2000): 303–309

2000: Shigeru Abe and Hiroko Ishizaki, Teikyo University, Fungus Research Center, "Infection Preventive Effect of Basidiomycetes Product AHCC on a Mouse Model with Opportunistic Infection," *Pharmacology Magazine* 12 (2000): 749–753

2000: R. Burikhanov, Dokkyo University, School of Medicine, et al., "Suppressive Effect of Active Hexose Correlated Compound (AHCC) on Thymic Apoptosis Induced by Dexamethasone in the Rat," *Endocrine Regulation* 34 (2000): 181–188

2000: Yasuo Kamiyama, Primary Surgery, Kansai Medical University, "AHCC (Active Hexose Correlated Compound) Usage Experience," *Biotherapy* 14, no. 10 (2000): 959–964

June 2001: Youichi Matsui, Primary Surgery, Kansai Medical University, "Effect on Preliminary Capacity of Liver by Administering AHCC As a Post Operative Supplementary Treatment for Liver Cell Cancer," Liver Cancer Society; and Konoe Chidzu, Kansai Medical University, Internal Medicine Department, "Prognosis Improvement Effect on Administering Functional Food (AHCC) As a Post Operative Supplementary Treatment for Liver Cell Cancer"

November 2001: 11th Convention of ASEAN Federation of Endocrine Societies, "Protective Effect of Basidiomycetes Culture Extract AHCC on Streptozotocin-Induced Diabetes and Chemical Substance Induced Thymic Apoptosis in the Rat," Amino Up Chemical Co. Ltd.

March 2002: Yasuo Kamiyama, Primary Surgery, Kansai Medical University, "Improved Prognosis of Postoperative Hepatocellular Carcinoma

Patients Treated with Functional Foods," *Journal of Hepatology* 37 (March 2002): 78–86

2002: Y. Matsui, et al., "Effect of AHCC on Gastric Cancer: Improved Prognosis of Postoperative Hepatocellular Carcinoma Patients When Treated with Functional Foods: A Prospective Cohort Study," *Journal of Hepatology* 37, no. 1 (2002): 78–86

2004: Hernan Aviles, Buxiang Sun, and Gerald Sonnenfeld, "Active Hexose Correlated Compound Enhances the Immune Function of Mice in the Hindlimb-Unloading Model of Spaceflight Conditions," *Journal of Applied Physiology* 97, no. 4 (2004): 1437–1444

2006: S. Cowawintaweewat, et al., "Prognostic Improvement of Patients with Advanced Liver Cancer after Active Hexose Correlated Compound (AHCC) treatment," *Asian Pacific Journal of Allergy & Immunology* 24 (2006): 34–45

2006: Y. Gao, D. Zhang, et al., "Active Hexose Correlated Compound Enhances Tumor Surveillance through Regulating Both Innate and Adaptive Immune Responses," *Cancer Immunology and Immunotherapy* 55, no. 10 (2006): 1258–1266

2007: H. Fujii, H. Nishioka, K. Wakame, and B. X. Sun, "Nutritional Food Active Hexose Correlated Compound (AHCC) Enhances Resistance against Bird Flu," *Japanese Journal of Complementary & Alternative Medicine* 1, no. 4 (2007): 37–39

2007: E. Spierings, H. Fujii, B. Sun, and T. Walshe, "A Phase I Study of the Safety of the Nutritional Supplement, Active Hexose Correlated Compound, AHCC, in Healthy Volunteers, *Journal of Nutrition, Science & Vitaminology* 53 (2007): 536–539

2008: C. Mach, H. Fujii, K. Wakame, and J. Smith, "Evaluation of Active Hexose Correlated Compound Hepatic Metabolism and Potential for Drug Interactions with Chemotherapy Agents," *Journal of Social & Integrative Oncology* 6, no. 3 (2008): 105–109

As mentioned above, there has been substantial medical research conducted on the effects of AHCC. There have been many more research reports besides those presented in this book, including research outside of Japan, in China, Korea, Thailand, and the United States.

ROLE OF AHCC
AS A SUPPLEMENTAL ALTERNATIVE MEDICINE

AHCC has been extensively researched and the number of doctors and health care professionals with a deeper understanding of AHCC has continued to increase. On the other hand, there are also many doctors who use only conventional pharmaceuticals and do not consider using alternative medicines. It is necessary to follow responsible medical protocols, but it is also important to respect the desires of the patient. Naturally, patients are not experts and ordinarily follow the recommendations of their physicians, but in certain circumstances, the doctor must consider what the patient wants.

The right to select the treatment method rests with the patient as long as there is informed consent. Therefore, in Japan, supplemental alternative medicines like AHCC are not discouraged as long as they are used at the urging of the patient, who agrees to take responsibility for the outcome. If AHCC is used, it must be adopted as a supplemental treatment by mutual consent of the doctor and the patient. Since it has been confirmed that there are no side effects of AHCC, there is no alteration of the intended effects of medical treatment. AHCC even demonstrates an ability to control side effects caused by anticancer drugs while enhancing efficacy.

ALTERNATIVE THERAPIES UNDER REVIEW
IN EUROPE AND AMERICA

The concept of immunotherapy—and especially cancer immunotherapy—has its roots in home remedies. Self-treatment has attracted more attention in recent years and has secured an important place in alternative medicine. Alternative treatments principally aim at restoring and building immunity. When a U.S. Senate Office of Technology Assessment report on alternative health care methods was published in 1990, Professor David Eisenberg of Harvard University conducted a survey of American citizens, using what were considered to be alternative treatments at the time. The results of this survey were published in the *New England Journal of Medicine* in 1993. According to the study, over 30 percent of Americans used complementary or alternative treatments at their own risk, in addition to or independent of prescriptions from their physicians. It was also reported that among the people who used alternative treatments, there was a high percentage of young and educated people. Before that, alternative therapies were considered nothing more than magic tricks used to cheat uneducated or elderly people and the prevailing wisdom was that they should be controlled. This was no less true in Japan and in Europe than it was in the United States.

The publication of Professor Eisenberg's research report was hailed as a turning point and a new approach to this issue began. The new thinking considered that the effects of home treatment and alternative practitioners could not be disregarded, but their safety and effectiveness should be medically tested. In 1992, the Office of Alternative Medicine (OAM) was established at the National Institutes of Health (NIH) in the United States. Beginning in 1993, health maintenance organizations (HMOs) in the United States began offering limited coverage of complementary and alternative treatments.

Among the 117 medical colleges whose responses were gathered in a 1998 survey related to complementary and alternative medicine (CAM) on CAM training and education in America, alternative medicine was introduced as an optional and sometimes compulsory subject in 75 medical schools. A similar survey was conducted in Japan that same year (at Jichi Medical School in Tsuruoka). In response to the query "Are treatments other than Western medicine—for example, Oriental medicine or home remedies—included in the lectures or practical training of medical students?" 18 out of 80 medical colleges across the country responded that "These subjects have been officially introduced."

In Japan, organizations like the Japanese Association for Alternative, Complementary and Traditional Medicine (JACT), the Japanese Institute of Complementary, Alternative Medicine (JCAM), and the Institute for Non-Pathological Systems were established in an effort to promote complementary and alternative medicine. Doctors and other health care professionals present papers and hold discussions on various types of alternative treatment and their ideal role in the future. Research results related to supplemental alternative treatments have been presented at academic conferences, and study sessions for AHCC have also been conducted at hospitals in Japan.

CHAPTER 2

AHCC in Cancer Treatment

AHCC has been used for the treatment of cancer in Japan, and has come to the fore as a health food that can be utilized for the purpose of prevention and amelioration of cancer as well. In the 1990s, AHCC monitoring tests were conducted. This was informal research in which cancer patients were given AHCC under the supervision of doctors and the effects were medically evaluated. This program became well-known because of the interest of the Japanese public in natural therapies.

A large amount of medical and pharmacological research took place. Clinical use increased, as it was voluntarily taken by cancer patients or recommended by their doctors. AHCC became trusted by experts as a health food that could be used as a supplement during cancer treatment. By the end of the 1990s, AHCC was known as a "health food for cancer" and used in as many as seven hundred medical institutions, including some outside of Japan. Unlike most health foods, which are primarily consumed as home remedies, AHCC has been used by doctors in the clinic and its effects have been medically and pharmacologically studied in detail.

In the United States, the Office of Alternative Medicine was established in 1992 at the National Institutes of Health (NIH), with the goal of researching alternative medicine. In the 1990s, the OTA (Office of Technology Assessment) of the U.S. Senate acknowledged the limitations of conventional cancer treatment, and published a report, titled "Unconventional Cancer Treatments" (GPO #052-003-01203-3), stating that further assessment of unconventional treatments (complementary and alternative) was necessary.

Cancer treatment falls into three main categories: surgery, chemotherapy, and radiotherapy. There are numerous problems with each of these types of treatment. For example, they are not effective for certain types of cancers or for cancer in advanced stages. They also incur severe side effects. Pharmacological and medical researchers are well aware of this, and many researchers are working specifically on the development of anticancer drugs without side effects. The common anticancer drugs today are toxic to cancer cells, but also to normal cells. This cell toxicity (known as cytotoxicity) acts specifically at the time of cell division. The drugs have a powerful effect on cancer cells, which proliferate by dividing with excessive frequency. However, many of the 60 trillion cells in our body—not just the cancer cells—are also undergoing division. Newly generated cells replace old cells in an ongoing cycle. Hair root cells, cells of the gastrointestinal tract, and blood cells are also cells in which the rate of division and replacement is particularly rapid, so these are especially vulnerable to anticancer drugs. The hair is not as significant, but the gastrointestinal tract and blood are fundamental systems that support vital activity. Therefore, important healthy cells are damaged by chemotherapy. Side effects of chemotherapy include hair loss, a decrease in the digestive absorption function as well as a decrease in the functioning of the whole body centered around the immune system, because of damage to blood cell production in the bone marrow.

AHCC: BECOMING RECOGNIZED AS A HEALTH FOOD FOR CANCER

Although the anticancer action expected from AHCC and the anticancer drugs are the same, their mechanisms of action are exactly the opposite. Part of the anticancer activity demonstrated by AHCC involves reviving the normal cells. Above all, AHCC has become recognized for its ability to activate the immune cells that destroy cancer cells, including white blood cells and lymphocytes. AHCC is also known for improving the body's inherent immunity. AHCC revives the body from its core, and there are no side effects from AHCC. AHCC is generally used as a supplemental treatment for many types of cancer and other medical problems (see Figure 2.1).

SPONTANEOUS REMISSION OF CANCER

It is medically recognized that spontaneous remission of cancer is possible, even if it is left untreated. From 1900 to 1965, U.S. medical scientists T. C. Everson and W. H. Cole (cited in *Spon-*

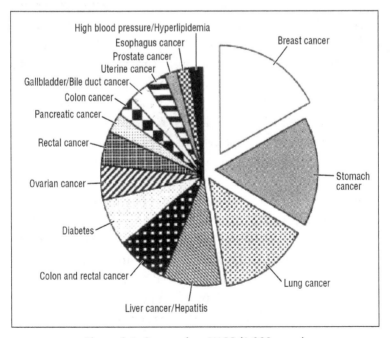

Figure 2.1 Cases using AHCC (1,000 cases)

taneous Regression of Cancer) collected and studied 176 examples of cases of natural spontaneous recovery among people with a confirmed diagnosis of cancer from all over the world. They concluded that the body can heal cancer on its own, even at an advanced stage.

Such natural recovery from cancer is medically regarded as exceptional. However, the relationship between immunity and cancer points up a possible mechanism explaining how this can happen. Immunotherapy is one way of assisting the body in self-recovery. The role of the immune system in cancer was powerfully illustrated in a discovery made on laboratory test mice at Wake Forest University. A biology professor named Zheng Cui was not a cancer researcher, but he used cancer cells on his test mice to extract antibodies from the abdominal fluid for his study on the metabolism of fats. He used a particularly virulent strain of cancer cells, called S180 cells, for this purpose. Usually, 200,000 cells caused death in all the mice within a month. A young researcher under Dr. Cui's supervision used this procedure on a new group of mice, but one mouse survived the injection of these virulent cells. She repeated the injection on this mouse without success. The next time she injected 2 million cells—ten times the normal dose! There was still no cancer and no abdominal swelling. This was unheard of, and Dr. Cui decided to administer the injection himself, this time an unprecedentedly high dose of 20 million S180 cancer cells. S180 cancer cells are usually so virulent that they destroy normal cells like wildfire. They proliferate so rapidly that in mice the tumor size doubles every ten hours. Yet two weeks after Dr. Cui himself injected the mice with 20 million S180 cancer cells, there was still no change. He then tried 200 million S180 cells—one thousand times the normal dose, but still no result. This mouse, which they named Mighty Mouse, was alive eight months later. Could this be an example of natural resistance to cancer? Could this lead to an explanation of the phenomenon of spontaneous remission?

The grandchildren of Mighty Mouse inherited this cancer immunity trait and allowed the researchers to continue to investigate this mysterious phenomenon. They were resistant even to 2 billion S180m cells, an injection of which comprised about 10 percent of their body weight. Imagine, as an analogy, a virulent tumor weighing 10 pounds being implanted into the body of a 100-pound woman! This is the burden that these mice were able to tolerate!

There was another surprise. After a delay of several months, these same mice inoculated with the cancer cells developed the abdominal swelling typical of tumor formation. Somehow they had all lost their incredible cancer resistance. Dr. Cui left them to die. Four weeks later when he returned, not only were they alive, but the swelling and all signs of the tumors were gone. He concluded that the resistance of the mice got weaker as they aged, but it was still strong enough to eventually overcome the burden of the injected cancer cells. After they recovered, they returned to robust health. The mystery of the fantastic cancer resistance was solved by Dr. Cui's colleague, Dr. Mark Miller, an expert on cancer cell development. Under microscopic examination he witnessed a powerful army of white blood cells attacking and ravaging the cancer cells instead of the other way around.

One of the body's most potent natural defenses is a type of white blood cell called the natural killer, or *NK* cell. These cells are sometimes called sentinel cells. They attack disease germs, virus-infected cells or abnormal incipient cancer cells. They attach to the abnormal cell or microbe and inject granules into them, causing them to rupture and break down into detritus that is then consumed by another type of white cell, called a macrophage. The granules inside the NK cells are constantly swirling, and this is an indicator of their activity. NK cell activity is an index of immune strength and is even used medically to determine the prognosis of cancer and AIDS patients. When NK cell activity is reduced to zero, death occurs. Measuring NK cell activity can help to accurately determine the number of months a patient has to live.

AHCC was discovered to increase NK cell activity. In as little as two weeks, NK cell activity can double or even triple, even in a sick person at an advanced stage of cancer. This property appears to have an additive effect on chemotherapy: Patients undergoing chemotherapy showed an enhanced response to treatment when they took AHCC. AHCC also promotes immune system modulation.

WHAT IS IMMUNITY?

The use of the word *immunity* is actually quite recent. *Immunity* in English is derived from the Latin word *immunitas*. In the Roman era, it was a word used in public administration to refer to exemption from taxes or public services. In the Middle Ages its meaning changed, and it came to refer to escaping from the epidemics of smallpox and black plague that were rampant in Europe. It was eventually adopted as a concept in medical science and medical treatment. *Immunity* indicates a series of mechanisms that help the body prevent and escape from infectious diseases. The basic concept of this mechanism is that living organisms discriminate between self and nonself, *defending* self from nonself. Immunology does not strictly see immunity as natural resistance against infection. Rather, it perceives immunity as the concept that living organisms differentiate the self from the surrounding environment and protect the integrity of the self throughout life.

HUMORAL IMMUNITY AND CELL-MEDIATED IMMUNITY

The immune system is complex, but scientists recognize two fundamental divisions within this system. These are *humoral immunity* and *cell-mediated* (or *cellular*) *immunity*.

Humoral Immunity

In the Black Plague epidemic of Europe in medieval times it was said that members of the clergy who survived did not get infected with Black Plague again, even if they were in close contact with victims. In 1700, Edward Jenner carried out the artificial inoculation of cowpox (bovine smallpox) virus and discovered that immunity against smallpox can be developed with the help of this artificial inoculation. In 1890, Emil von Behring and Shibasaburo Kitazato discovered the immunotoxin. They reported the presence of a substance that specifically neutralized the toxin in the blood of animals that were injected with toxin-producing bacteria, such as diphtheria or tetanus. They proved that this substance was found in the "humoral" (fluid) component of the blood, or the serum. When this serum was administered, it had a dramatic effect on the patients afflicted with diphtheria and tetanus. This marked the beginning of what is known as serum treatment. Later on, this substance was called an *anti-*

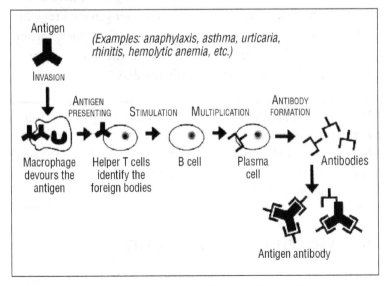

Figure 2.2 Mechanism of humoral immunity

body and was found to be a protein. Likewise, the foreign body of microbial origin that induces antibody formation is called an *antigen* (see Figure 2.2 on page 29).

Cell-Mediated Immunity

The humoral substance, known as the antibody, which neutralizes the toxin, was considered to provide the real immunity. In the second half of the nineteenth century, a theory emerged that the cell produces the antibody and is the actual provider of immunity. This was called the cell theory, in opposition to the above-mentioned humoral theory of immunity.

According to the Russian bacteriologist Elie Metchnikov, white blood cells taken from infected living organisms (particularly macrophages) have a strong capacity to kill pathogenic microbes by engulfing and destroying the pathogens. From this beginning point, Metchnikov discovered various reactions that occur without recourse to antibodies, such as delayed allergy, graft-rejection reactions, contact hypersensitivity, target cell destruction by lymphocytes, and the like, which were later grouped together under the heading of cell-mediated immunity. This phenomenon of cell-mediated immunity was considered the main sphere of immunology in modern times (see Figure 2.3).

The immunocompetent cells that participate actively in cell-mediated immunity intercommunicate through transmitter substances between these cells. These chemical messengers, such as cytokines and lymphokines, are proteins that control the immune system by transmitting information between cells.

AHCC AND CELL-MEDIATED IMMUNITY

AHCC stimulates (or modulates) cell-mediated immunity by activating the white blood cells and lymphocytes that directly attack

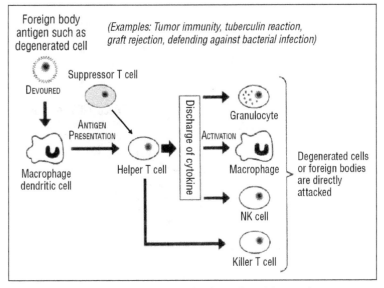

Figure 2.3 Mechanism of cell-mediated immunity

abnormal cells, virus-infected cells or external viral and bacterial pathogens that enter the body. AHCC does not destroy cancer cells directly, as in the case of anticancer drugs, but fights against cancer indirectly by stimulating the immunocompetent cells and fortifying the body's natural response.

IMMUNITY AND DISEASE

The relationship between immunity and conditions related to lifestyle, such as diabetes, high blood pressure, arteriosclerosis, hyperlipidemia, and the like remained unnoticed until recently. If we look at the cause of chronic diseases from the standpoint of their relationship to the hypofunctioning of various internal organs and blood vessels, we can see that there may be some immune cells in the structure of these organs that cannot fulfill the normal functions.

The network of the nervous system, the immune system, and the endocrine system interact together as the fundamental con-

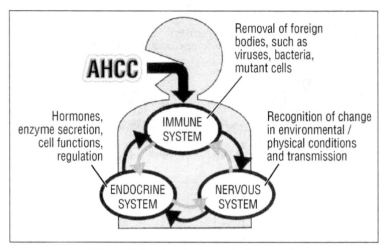

Figure 2.4 Living body control network

trol system of the body, rather than the internal organs or cells of the body. There is a possibility of hidden disease if any abnormality is generated within the immune system (see Figure 2.4).

AHCC activates cell-mediated immunity and simultaneously affects all body functions. It can also assist in the prevention and cure of lifestyle-related diseases. The old Chinese medical concept of curing the sick *person*—rather than the sickness—is now being reexamined in light of alternative treatments, such as health foods and dietary supplements.

According to the published data, cited on pages 16–19, AHCC has an antineoplastic effect (that is, it prevents abnormal growth), an anti-diabetic effect, an antihepatitis effect, an anti-inflammatory effect, and a tranquilizing effect. These effects do not contradict each other but, rather, contribute to adjusting the balance of the entire body.

MUSHROOMS AND IMMUNITY

It has been said that shiitake mushrooms are effective against cancer and that cancer can be cured by taking reishi mushrooms.

There have been reports of tumor reduction and even cures of cancer using Chinese medicines or home remedies. It has been observed that these traditional remedies work by activating the natural healing power, or the inherent immunity, of the patient. Mushroom-based immunostimulant products were developed with the aim of using them in cancer treatment.

Constituents isolated from mushrooms have not only been certified as medicines in Japan, but are also recognized as having immunostimulating and antineoplastic effects. Lentinan and Krestin are representative examples. They are recognized as anticancer agents in modern medicine as well. These medicines are not to be taken alone, but can be used effectively when taken with anticancer drugs in hospitals (see Table 2.1).

TABLE 2.1 MUSHROOM-BASED ANTINEOPLASTIC AGENTS

ELEMENT Medicine	ORIGIN	POTENCY AND EFFECTS
Lentinan	Shiitake carpophores (fruiting bodies)	β-(1,6)-branched β-(1,3)-glucan. Extension of survival time in patients with nonoperable cancers or who have recurrent stomach cancer; oral administration of this medicine concomitant with tegafur.
Schizophiran	Suehirotake culture filtrate	β-(1,6)-branched β-(1,3)-glucan. Reinforcement of direct effect of radiation therapy in cervical cancer.
Krestin	Kawaratake mycelium	β-glucan bounded with protein. Extension of survival time by using this drug with chemotherapy in stomach cancer and colorectal cancer. Prolonged period of health when used with chemotherapy for small-cell lung cancer.

AHCC AND IMMUNE MECHANISMS

White blood cells (leukocytes) are the main immunocompetent cells. There are different types of white blood cells: neutrophils, eosinophils, basophils, macrophages, B lymphocytes (B cells), and thymus-dependent lymphocytes (T cells). All these cells are interrelated and coordinate within the body to form our cellular (cell-mediated) immunity mechanism. The cell-mediated immune system is particularly important for protection from the chronic diseases that we are subject to after maturity. The humoral immune system is important in childhood and manufactures antibodies to various diseases, but it is helpless in combating the more chronic diseases. Many people have antibodies to herpes virus, for example, but the presence of antibodies does not mean there is immunity. Likewise, detection of antibodies to the AIDS virus are how the presence of HIV is diagnosed. The cell-mediated immune system, by contrast, has the mechanisms that can actually heal a disease and engineer a spontaneous remission. Other white blood cells include natural killer (NK) cells, mentioned earlier, and cytotoxic T cells (killer T cells). A lot of information has been derived from examining the blood of cancer patients to elucidate some of the immune mechanisms and the effects of AHCC.

ACTIVITY OF HELPER T CELLS IS THE KEY TO CELL-MEDIATED IMMUNITY

There are several types of T (thymus-dependent) cells. One type is called the *helper T cell*. There are three types of helper T cells, as shown below.

1. Helper T0 type (also known as Th0/Helper T naive cells)

2. Helper T1 type (Th1) cellular immunity

3. Helper T2 type (Th2) humoral immunity

Th1 and Th2 are formed from the cell differentiation of T0 cells. On receiving a chemical signal, helper T cells promote the differentiation from Th0 to Th1 and there is an increase in the number of Th1 cells activated among the helper T cells. At the same time, the Th1 cells send a communication for activating the killer T cells (cytotoxic T lymphocytes, or CTL) and lymphokine-activated killer (LAK) cells that launch a full-scale attack on cancer cells. This is the broad role of the helper T cells in cell-mediated immunity.

> The LAK cells are activated by a cytokine called *interleukin-2* (IL-2), which is produced by helper T cells, and these LAK cells attack cancer cells by secreting a substance called *perforin*.

If we examine the blood of cancer patients who are taking AHCC, it has been confirmed that it contains more Th1 cells than Th2 cells. A chemical messenger (cytokine) that activates the killer T cells is discharged from macrophages, or Th1 cells, in the bodies of patients who are taking AHCC. As a result, the cell-mediated immunity is improved. Interferon is the most famous cytokine. There are also cytokines called *interleukins* and various *factors*, such as tumor necrosis factor, that transmit information on how to handle a potential threat to the cellular environment.

> In the early years of the AIDS epidemic, it was discovered that there were hundreds of people who were HIV-positive, but perfectly healthy, showing no signs of the disease. Further investigation determined that HIV+ people with no disease were those with active cell-mediated immunity (Th1), while HIV+ people whose immune systems were biased toward humoral immunity (Th2) manifested AIDS. Expression of cell-mediated immunity is necessary both for the prevention and successful treatment of chronic degenerative diseases.

THE ROLE OF CYTOKINES IN IMMUNE STRENGTH

Cytokines are chemical messengers released from immunocytes. In this way they play a role that is similar to the role played by hormones in the endocrine system. Cytokines mediate the interaction between cells concerned with immune reactions, which is why some of them are called interleukins. They communicate between leukocytes (white blood cells). Interferon (IFN) interferes with viral activity, tumor necrosis factor (TNF) breaks down tumors, colony-stimulating factor (CSF) stimulates white blood cell formation, and erythropoietin (EPO) stimulates red blood cell formation. Almost all malignancies are associated with suppression of cell-mediated immunity. Some of the cytokines that activate cell-mediated immunity and enhance the body's ability to attack cancer cells, are shown in Table 2.2.

TABLE 2.2 MUSHROOM-BASED ANTITUMOR SUBSTANCES

CYTOKINE	MAIN FUNCTION
TNF-α; Tumor necrosis factor alpha	Inducing IL-1, inducing GM-CSF, cytotoxic and cytostatic activity, inducing IFN-γ secretion
IFN-γ; Gamma interferon	Macrophage activation; NK cell activation
IL-2; Interleukin 2	Inducing T cell proliferation/differentiation, NK cell proliferation/activation, LAK cells, macrophage activation
IL-12; Interleukin 12	Inducing IFN-γ production by activating NK cells; inducing differentiation of Th0 to Th1
IL-18; Interleukin 18	Inducing IFN-γ production; lymphocyte activation

SCIENTIFICALLY ANALYZING IMMUNE COMPETENCE

Natural killer (NK) cells are of primary importance. NK cells first detect and fight abnormal cells, including cancer cells. NK cell activity is a vital factor in cancer immunotherapy. Nevertheless, there have been recent reports of development of cancer in patients with high NK cell activity. Analysis of a large volume of statistical data was needed to interpret this phenomenon. Dr. Katsuaki Uno, chief director of Comfort Hospital in Yokohama, has analyzed this information according to a system of blood analysis that he developed called the cancer immunity screening. With this tool, he has discovered the role of several other key factors in cancer development involving the immune system.

When we consider the role of the immune system with respect to cancer proliferation, we must bear in mind that the macrophages that capture the substances discharged into the body fluid from the cancer cells (cancer antigen peptides) secrete interleukin-12. This cytokine stimulates the helper T cells (Th0) and promotes their differentiation into helper T1 cells (Th1). The activated Th1 cells release gamma interferon (IFN-γ) and activate NK cells and LAK cells. These cells are immune cells, which attack the cancer cells.

Since there is a proliferation of cancer cells in cancer patients, immunosuppressive agents are produced and macrophage activity is suppressed; therefore, interleukin-12 production is weak. The Th0 cells differentiate into helper Th2-type cells that suppress immune competence; cytokines like transforming growth factor (TGF-β) are then produced. Consequently, cancer patients do not have sufficient immune strength to overcome cancer and the proliferation of cancer cells is accelerated (see Figure 2.5). The immune system is biased away from cell-mediated immunity toward humoral immunity, which only addresses short-term acute problems.

By contrast, cytokines like TNF-α, IFN-γ, and interleukin-12 (IL-12) are actively produced in patients who take AHCC, and it is believed that this stops or reduces the proliferation of the tumor (see Figure 2.6). Blood tests show an increase in these markers of immune competence.

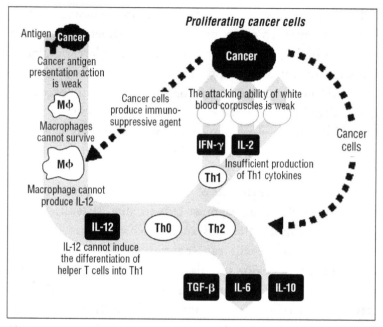

Figure 2.5 Suppression of tumor immunity in the tumor-bearing state

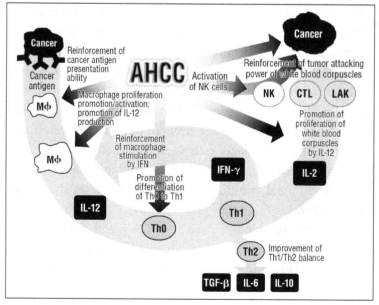

Figure 2.6 Promotion of tumor immunity with AHCC

CLINICALLY APPLICABLE IMMUNOLOGICAL TESTS

Dr. Katsuaki Uno of Comfort Hospital has set up a tumor immunity outpatient clinic at Comfort Hospital and has established a technique of numerically analyzing the changes in the immunity mechanisms affected by the development or progression of cancer as immunity parameters. He has also used this information to develop his method of cancer immunity screening. Dr. Uno's research findings, based on the data obtained from this cancer immunity screening and the effects of AHCC on cell-mediated immunity, have also been confirmed.

Figure 2.7 compares the capacity of 172 healthy people and 567 cancer patients to produce IL-12 and IFN-γ. The graph on the left shows IL-12–producing capacity. The average is close to 30 and the maximum has crossed 40 in healthy people. However, it is concentrated around a low level that does not even reach 10 in cancer patients. There is no stimulation for differentiation/maturation of white cells from Th0 to Th1 in an immune environment in which IL-12 is insufficient. In a low-activity immune environment, in which Th1 is reduced, there is a short supply of

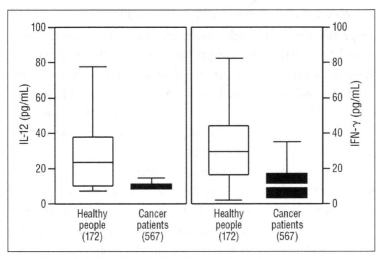

Figure 2.7 Cytokines in healthy people and cancer patients

IFN-γ and there is no increase in the count or the activity of the killer T cells.

The graph on the right in Figure 2.7 shows the IFN-γ-producing capacity. The average is close to 30 in healthy people. However, the average is less than 10 and the maximum level does not even reach 20 in cancer patients. The cytotoxic T cell (killer T cell) count decreases and its activity is also low when IFN-γ is insufficient. The result is that cancer cells are overlooked and proliferate, instead of being eliminated.

When NK cell activation was compared, it was also found that NK cell activation is higher in people with cancer than healthy people. This does not mean that there is cancer because NK cell activation is high. Rather, it can be interpreted that there is an increase in NK activity as a result of cancer.

AHCC INCREASES THE PRODUCTION OF CYTOKINES THAT ACTIVATE CELL-MEDIATED IMMUNITY

If we sequentially follow the diagram, a deeper understanding on the background of the immune activity is gained when AHCC is in use.

Figure 2.8 summarizes the data obtained by Dr. Uno with the cooperation of thirty-eight cancer patients who had come for a consultation. These thirty-eight people were medically diagnosed as having stage IV cancer and were in a so-called "terminal stage" of cancer and believed to have been given up on by their doctors. Dr. Uno prescribed 6g of AHCC per day, divided equally into three portions to all of these patients, and then observed the amounts of cytokines produced.

Figure 2.8 shows the change in the amount of IL-12 produced. Although the production capacity was centered at a low level of around 10 before taking AHCC, there was a notable increase in the second month from the beginning of intake of AHCC. By the fourth month the levels approached the levels of healthy people. This indicated that there was a rise in the Th1 count and its acti-

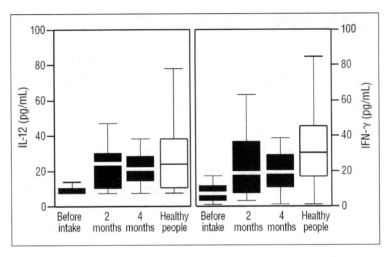

Figure 2.8 Quantities of cytokines produced in cancer patients
taking AHCC

vation with the intake of AHCC. It also indicated that there were
a few cases in which there was no rise in the amount of IL-12
production, despite the fact that AHCC was taken.

Table 2.3 shows the change in the level of IFN-γ produced.
Although the production capacity was centered at around 10
before taking AHCC, there was a definite rise in the production
capacity in the fourth month after starting AHCC. There is a cor-
responding increase in the count as well as in the *activity* of the
killer T cells as IFN-γ production increases. So activation of Th1
immunity working with the killer T cells enhances the ability to
fight even advanced stages of cancer.

Table 2.3 is a summary of the interaction of IL-12 and
IFN-γ produced after starting AHCC. Ninety percent of the people who had excellent IL-12 as well as IFN-γ production were
found to be in good health. On the other hand, satisfactory treatment results were not observed in patients having insufficient
production of either one of the cytokines. The combined activities of IL-12 and IFN-γ demonstrated a synergy in developing a
high capacity to produce Th1 cytokines.

TABLE 2.3 TH1-RELATED CYTOKINE INTERACTION		
	Group with good IL-12	Group with bad IL-12
Group with good IFN-γ	90.0%	66.0%
Group with bad IFN-γ	25.0%	8.5%

It is clear from these findings that AHCC exhibits a strong effect in enhancing cell-mediated immunity in most of the cases. Naturally, there are some exceptions, but overall a positive effect can be expected.

Refer to Table 2.4 for the immunological tests used.

TABLE 2.4 IMMUNOLOGICAL TESTS FOR CANCER	
CELL-MEDIATED IMMUNITY TESTS	CANCER STATUS CHECKS
Cytokine tests IL-12 IFN-γ TNF-α	Important activators released from immune cells, such as lymphocytes and macrophages, for monitoring cancer progression.
Helper T cell classification tests Th1 type Th2 type Th1/Th2 ratio	Th1 immune cells work to suppress the growth of cancer. Conversely, Th2 are immune cells that promote the growth of cancer. The balance of immunity can be assessed with this ratio.
Cytotoxic activation test NK cell activity	Cells that increase the degree of activity against cancer generation and attack cancer cells. Test to check whether the degree of activity is increased for some reason.
Cancer-relevant antigen test CEA, AFP, CA 19-9, DUPAN-2 and other 20 types	Substances that increase at the appearance and growth of cancer and are detected as foreign bodies by the immune system; they are also considered tumor markers. Early detection is useful for diagnosis.

FUNCTIONAL FOODS ARE NOT THE ONLY WAY TO STRENGTHEN IMMUNITY

Dr. Max Gerson (1881–1951), known throughout the world for his diet therapy for cancer, proved in numerous cases that many kinds of cancer can be cured by increasing the immune strength through a comprehensive diet and internal cleansing therapy. The Simonton Method and Meaningful Life Therapy, based on the work of O. Carl Simonton, suggests the possibility of recovering from cancer by increasing immune strength by means of a psychologically supportive approach.

The notion that cancer can be cured if stress on the body from the accumulation of undesirable diet or psychological influences can be eliminated or controlled has been in existence since ancient times and is now being advocated again by many experts. Research has been conducted into the relationship between psychological condition and disease. Data has been published on epidemiological research into health psychology, suggesting that there is a high risk of cancer in people who are under high internal stress.

Breath control and psychological approaches, such as meditation or psychological counseling, are also excellent ways to increase immune strength. Aromatherapy, using aromatic essential oils, provides beneficial psychological effects in addition to reducing pain and ameliorating other symptoms. Scientific data concerning the results of these methods will be explored in the future.

AHCC is certainly one way of strengthening cell-mediated immunity. However, AHCC by itself is not sufficient. It is crucial to reduce the stress on the body caused by eating habits, lifestyle, and the environment in order to continue on the path to recovery.

FURTHER PROOF OF IMMUNE ACTIVITY

Numerous basic research studies show that AHCC improves the immunity of living organisms through several mechanisms:

- It induces the production of cytokines that reinforce cellular immunity, such as TNF-α, IFN-γ, IL-1, IL-2, etc.

- It activates immune cells that attack cancer cells, such as macrophages, NK cells, LAK cells, killer T cells, etc.

- It reinforces the activity of Th1 immune cells (helper Th1 type cells), necessary for the activation of cellular immunity.

- It suppresses the production of cytokines, such as TGF-β, which inhibit cellular immunity.

Which component of AHCC acts in what way has not yet been clarified. However, it is known that polysaccharides work through various mechanisms to improve vital function and energy with a focus on immunity. This is an important point. AHCC, as well as all health foods, are effective not for one particular part of the body, but for the body as a whole.

ACTIVATION OF NEUTROPHILS AND MACROPHAGES BY AHCC

Stimulation of neutrophils and macrophages, which are types of white blood cells, is vital in the initial stages of activation of cellular immunity. In the case of actual injury, the role of neutrophils and macrophages is to fight external invaders (for example, bacteria), which quickly collect on a wound. Cellular immunity begins when the neutrophils and macrophages are activated. In some cases, the resistance of the immune system is accompanied by a severe inflammatory reaction, such as a fever. Professor Masatoshi Yamazaki of the Department of Pharmacology, Teikyo University, observed that AHCC activated these white blood cells and conducted experiments based on his discovery.

• Cumulative action of neutrophils. When AHCC is injected in the abdominal cavity (peritoneum) of test mice, white blood cells (especially neutrophils) in the abdominal cavity are activated and accumulate to fight the infection. The cellular-immunity stimulation from AHCC is measured by counting the number of neutrophils. When AHCC was administered intraperitoneally and the number of accumulated cells was counted, it was confirmed that 80 percent of the accumulated cells were neutrophils. The higher the value, the higher the level of white blood cell stimulation. Moreover, when these neutrophils were examined, it was found that they released a protein called calprotectin, which has a strong cancer-destroying effect.

• Action on mouse MM46 breast cancer model. Breast cancer was transplanted into mice and then AHCC (20mg) injected intraperitoneally. After one month, the size of the tumor had shrunk up to 60 percent, compared to a group that did not receive AHCC (see Figure 2.9). In the AHCC-administered mice, the presence of TNF-α was confirmed, in addition to calprotectin. TNF-α is mainly produced by the macrophages; therefore, it was assumed that the cancer cells were attacked by the macrophages and killed by the TNF-α produced by them (see Figure 2.10).

PRODUCTION OF IL-12 BY MACROPHAGES AFTER ADMINISTRATION OF AHCC

IL-12 (interleukin-12) is a cytokine produced by macrophages or lymphocytes. It is a key factor in sustaining and activating immunity. A group of doctors, led by Nobuo Takemori of Asahigawa Public Service Hospital, conducted experiments using mice to confirm whether IL-12 is produced from stimulation of macrophages with AHCC. AHCC was injected into the abdomen of the mice and changes in the "milky spots" of the dor-

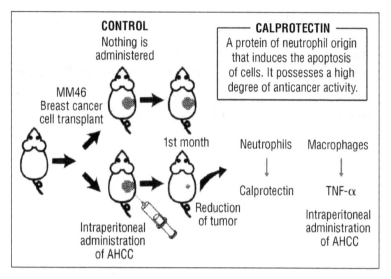

Figure 2.9 Effect of AHCC on the cell-damaging action of calprotectin

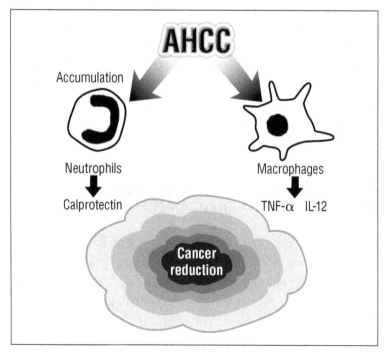

Figure 2.10 Cancer-killing action of neutrophils and macrophages

sal mesogastrium, or omentum, the region where macrophages and lymphocytes are produced, were observed with an electron microscope. In mice given AHCC, a large volume of IL-12–positive macrophages in various stages of differentiation appeared in the omental milky spots. It is clear that AHCC significantly induces differentiation and growth of macrophages, and it also increases the IL-12–producing ability of macrophages. The ability of macrophages to produce cytokines (IL-12, IFN-γ, TNF-α) is measured to check the quality of AHCC at Amino Up Co. Ltd., the manufacturer of AHCC. Testing for these cytokines is an important indicator for measuring the actual immunocompetence of a cancer patient with a blood test.

CONFIRMATION OF CYTOKINE-PRODUCING ABILITY BY THE LOW MOLECULAR WEIGHT POLYSACCHARIDES OF AHCC

The Cancer Research Unit of the Pathology Division of the Department of Medicine, Hokkaido University, played a central role in this research. Each element of AHCC was divided into high molecular weight (like β-glucans) and low molecular weight (like α-glucans) components by the column-separation method. Experiments were carried out using cancer-bearing mice. When the lung cells of AHCC-administered cancer-bearing mice were examined, it was seen that both IL-12 and TNF-α were strongly induced, but induction of IL-12 was strongest when the low molecular weight components were administered. Moreover, both the high molecular weight and low molecular weight components of AHCC controlled the production of TGF-β, which is an immunosuppressive cytokine (see Table 2.5).

It is known that the low molecular weight polysaccharides (molecular weight 5,000 daltons) of AHCC are primarily effective in improving the production capability of cytokines with immunostimulating action.

			LOW MOLECULAR WEIGHT	HIGH MOLECULAR WEIGHT
CYTOKINE	CONTROL	AHCC	COMPONENT	COMPONENT
TABLE 2.5 MANIFESTATION OF CYTOKINES IN MICE HAVING CANCER BY AHCC ACCORDING TO ITS COMPONENTS				
Spleen cells				
IL-2	Not detected	**Remarkable manifestation**	Moderate manifestation	Moderate manifestation
IL-12	Not detected	Moderate manifestation	**Remarkable manifestation**	Not detected
TNF-α	Not detected	**Remarkable manifestation**	Moderate manifestation	Moderate manifestation
Tumor formation				
TGF-β	**Remarkable manifestation**	Not detected	Not detected	Not detected

AHCC IMPROVES IMMUNE SURVEILLANCE

Immune surveillance is the function of the immune system to discover the presence of cancer development in the body. Cancer cells have mechanisms they use to hide their presence and escape detection by the immune system. Researchers at Yale University and Amino Up Chemical Company in Japan tested the effect of AHCC on immune surveillance in cancer. Reactivating immune surveillance means that tumor cells can be unmasked. Then the immune system is able once again to detect and destroy them. White blood cells and the interferon they secrete are necessary for the immune system to be able to detect tumors. In test animals, oral administration of AHCC significantly delayed melanoma formation and reduced tumor size. They found that AHCC significantly increased tumor-antigen-specific immune cells and their ability to produce interferon (gamma interferon: IFN-γ). The researchers indicated that there are a number of possible ways that AHCC could accomplish this, but the important fact is that their research confirms the tumor-reducing ability of AHCC through another immune mechanism.

AHCC REDUCES THE SIDE EFFECTS OF ANTICANCER DRUGS

There is a wide range of side effects caused by anticancer drugs (chemotherapy drugs), such as nausea, vomiting, hair loss, loss of appetite, impaired liver function, leukopenia (low white cell count), thrombocytopenia (low platelet count), and anemia. Not only do these drugs cause severe pain, but they can also decrease immunity and vital energy. AHCC is known to be very effective in reducing the side effects of anticancer drugs. This has been observed in a number of cases of cancer patients who were taking AHCC with chemotherapy. It has also been observed in animal tests. The use of AHCC with chemotherapy not only reduces the side effects of anticancer drugs but also maximizes their cancer-destroying activity. Although it depends on the type of drug and the type of cancer, good treatment results can usually be achieved through the combination of a low-dose chemotherapy and AHCC.

LIFE-EXTENDING ACTIVITY OF AHCC WITH CHEMOTHERAPY

Professor Masumi Hosokawa, of the Pathology Department of the Cancer Research Institute (now the Genetic Disease Research Institute) of Hokkaido University, combined small doses of low-dose chemotherapy and AHCC and examined whether it had a life-extending effect on rats with a type of breast cancer that metastasizes easily (see Figure 2.11). He confirmed the life-prolonging effect of using the anticancer drug cyclophosphamide (CY) and AHCC in combination.

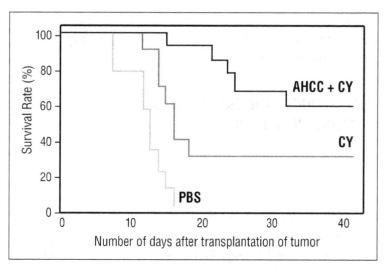

Figure 2.11 Combined effects of CY and AHCC on rats
with breast cancer

Professor Hosokawa also discovered that the NK activity suppressed by the anticancer drug UFT was restored when AHCC was used concomitantly. It was also found that lymph-node metastases from the breast tumors were significantly suppressed by the simultaneous use of AHCC. Even though anticancer drugs generally have a frightening reputation for causing severe side effects, they can be effectively used by skillfully combining them with immunostimulants, depending on the type and stage of the cancer. According to Professor Hosokawa, it is possible to maximize the good points of the anticancer drugs and AHCC with combined use of small doses of the anticancer drug with the immunostimulating properties of AHCC.

AHCC PREVENTS HAIR LOSS FROM CHEMOTHERAPY

Hair loss is a frequent side effect of chemotherapy. Many doctors have reported that AHCC prevents chemotherapy-related hair loss. Because of these reports, researchers at Amino Up decided to study it with an animal-test model. Eight-day-old rats were divided into groups. Each group was subjected to one of the following conditions:

Group 1: Bred normally for comparative study (control group)

Group 2: Given 30mg/kg per day of the anticancer drug (cytosine arabinoside = Ara-C) for seven days.

Group 3: Given 500mg/kg per day of AHCC orally along with the same anticancer drug as Group 2

In the case of Group 2, the hair loss began the fifth day after first taking the drug; a high rate of hair loss was seen in five of the seven rats by the ninth day. Hair loss prevention was clearly recognized in the group in which AHCC was administered concomitantly. The rate of hair loss in six of the nine rats was less than 25 percent (see Table 2.6). Needless to say, the results of the animal tests are not necessarily reflected in humans. However, if the many reported cases of this effect are combined, it can be said that hair loss as a side effect of chemotherapy is suppressed to a considerable degree by AHCC.

TABLE 2.6 EFFECT OF AHCC ON ARA-C INDUCED DEPILATION

	NUMBER OF RATS	DEGREE OF HAIR LOSS			
		NONE	LOW	MEDIUM	HEAVY
Control	3	3	0	0	0
Ara-C	7	0	1	1	5
Ara-C + AHCC	9	4	2	2	1

MYELOSUPPRESSION FROM CHEMOTHERAPY PREVENTED BY AHCC

Since anticancer drugs suppress the function of the bone marrow, which is the blood cell "production factory," chemotherapy can lead to a decrease in both the white and red blood cell counts. This side effect is known as *myelosuppression*.

Bone marrow is a cavernous, spongy, hematopoietic (blood cell–producing) tissue inside the bones. White blood cells, red blood cells, and platelets are continuously formed there. The bone marrow contains the myeloid stem cells (hematopoietic stem cells) that are the starting point of blood cells. Red blood cells transport oxygen and white blood cells fight bacteria that invade from outside. Platelets stop bleeding. These blood cells are all formed in the bone marrow and then discharged into the blood.

Myelosuppression is a dangerous side effect, because if cancer patients have low red cell counts, they are anemic and the resulting fatigue weakens their overall condition. If the white blood cell counts are low, the immune system is weak and they are vulnerable to potentially fatal infections. Many doctors who carry out clinical tests have already reported reduction in myelosuppression in cancer patients who are taking AHCC during chemotherapy. Dr. G. H. Ahn of Ok-Cherm Hospital in South Korea has reported that there was a definite increase in the white blood cell count in a total of twelve cancer patients suffering from stage III–IV cancer (two patients each with breast cancer, stomach cancer, lung cancer, liver cancer, uterine cancer, and ovarian cancer) who were taking 6g of AHCC per day, as shown in Figure 2.12.

Animal studies have also shown a reduction in damage to the marrow of mice who were administered AHCC along with chemotherapy. The anticancer drugs used in these tests were fluorouracil (5-FU) and cyclophosphamide (CY). As seen in Figure 2.13, the red blood cell count was maintained at a level close to normal in the mice that received AHCC along with the anticancer drugs (5-FU + AHCC group and CY + AHCC group). Of course, there were also some cases in which there was no tumor (cancer) reduction effect from AHCC. However, AHCC reduced the burden on the patients by reducing the side effects of chemotherapy. This observation is supported by numerous studies.

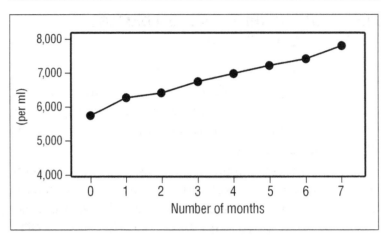

Figure 2.12 Change in white blood cell count of
AHCC-administered cancer patients

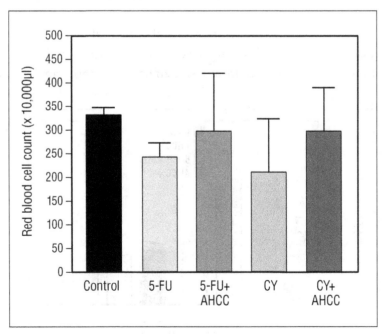

Figure 2.13 Effect of AHCC on myelosuppression
caused by anticancer drugs

AHCC PROTECTS THE LIVER FROM DAMAGE CAUSED BY CHEMOTHERAPY

The liver is responsible for the detoxification of poisonous substances (including drugs). The heavier the toxic burden, the more damage is caused to the liver. This organ is damaged significantly by chemotherapy. Liver failure is one of the most dangerous side effects of anticancer drugs.

When AHCC was administered along with the anticancer drugs mercaptopurine (6-MP) and methotrexate (MTX) in mice, the result shown in Figure 2.14 was obtained after liver function failure was observed. The values of both liver enzymes GOT and GPT in the serum (which are the indices of liver function failure) were almost normal in the mice given AHCC along with the anticancer drugs. The numerical values of the liver enzymes were extremely high in the case of mice that were given only the anticancer drugs.

AHCC also works for the recovery and support of liver function. It is not limited to mitigating the effects of liver function failure; it also prevents liver failure as a side effect of chemotherapy.

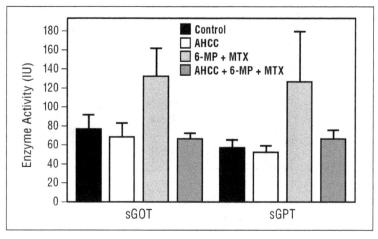

Figure 2.14 Effect of AHCC on serum liver enzyme levels in mice with chemotherapy-induced liver damage

CHAPTER 3

Effects of AHCC
on Other Diseases

Much of the research into the effects of AHCC has been conducted in Japan. In recent years more research has been conducted in other countries, including the United States, at the University of California at Davis, Yale University, M.D. Anderson Research Center at the University of Texas, and other venues. There are also a growing number of clinicians using AHCC in day-to-day medical practice. Dr. Dan Kenner of California conducted an informal survey of doctors in the United States who used large quantities of AHCC in their clinical practices. In addition to using AHCC for treating cancer, there is also an increase in its use for type C hepatitis. One doctor who is a pain specialist pointed out that many patients addicted to methadone develop hepatitis. He uses AHCC in 4.5g daily doses and reduced the viral load in over half of the hepatitis C patients using methadone, sometimes even down to an undetectable level. Other clinical applications mentioned include chronic fatigue syndrome, which is often a viral disorder. Allergic rhinitis (hay fever), chronic sinus infections, pediatric respiratory infections, eczema, colds, and flu are other complaints that doctors are beginning to address with AHCC. Some doctors have recommended AHCC for post-traumatic stress disorder (PSTD) and have used it to protect NK cell activity, since NK cell activity is reduced by stress and trauma. Even military personnel with severe cases of PTSD have had their symptoms ameliorated by AHCC: Not only have they seen improvement in their general health, but they have also experienced a moderation in their stress-related symptoms.

EFFECT ON DIABETES DISCOVERED IN BASIC RESEARCH

Diabetes is caused by a shortage of insulin produced by the pancreas (type 1) or by metabolic hyposensitivity (slow reaction) to insulin (type 2). As a result, it is a chronic disease in which the blood sugar level rises because the glucose in the blood cannot be metabolized. There have been reports of cases of a decline in the blood sugar levels of diabetic patients and an alleviation of complications as a result of patients taking AHCC. There has also been clear evidence of preventive effects of AHCC with regard to type 1 diabetes in animal tests. The rise in blood sugar levels in rats was suppressed upon administration of AHCC, as shown in Figure 3.1.

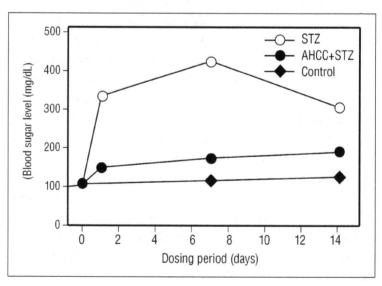

Figure 3.1 Effect of AHCC on STZ-induced diabetes

Group 1: Bred normally for comparative study (control group)

Group 2: Diabetic model with pancreatic failure induced by administration of streptozotocin (STZ)

Group 3: Given 3 percent AHCC liquid solution orally, in advance, along with STZ

The three groups were observed for two weeks and compared. There was an increase in the weight of the control group (Group 1), whereas weight reduction as well as deterioration in the coat were seen in the diabetic model Group 2. Although a slight rise was observed in the blood sugar levels of diabetic model Group 3, which was coadministered AHCC, the levels remained within the normal range and weight reduction was also controlled. When the pancreatic tissues were inspected with a microscope, damaged islets of Langerhans, the insulin-producing cells, were observed in the diabetic-model rats, whereas cell damage to the islets was prevented in the group that was given AHCC. This suggests that AHCC protects the insulin-producing cells and normalizes insulin production.

EFFECT OF AHCC ON A LIVER-DAMAGED MOUSE MODEL

AHCC was administered in advance to mice that were subsequently treated with carbon tetrachloride to induce liver damage. AHCC prevented a decrease in the detoxification metabolic enzyme glutathione S-transferase (GST) in the liver. Moreover, when the liver cells were observed under a microscope, it was found that cell destruction had also been prevented (see Figure 3.2). As a result, it became apparent that AHCC prevented liver damage caused by the oxidation due to a toxic substance like carbon tetrachloride.

When a lot of liver cells are destroyed by fulminant hepatic failure (severe impairment of liver function in the absence of pre-

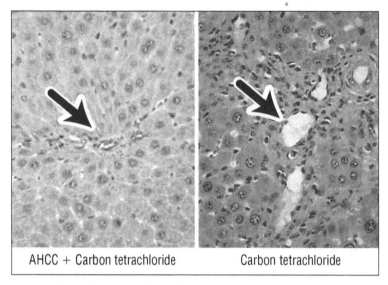

| AHCC + Carbon tetrachloride | Carbon tetrachloride |

Figure 3.2 Prevention of hepatic cell necrosis by AHCC

existing liver disease), the rate of fatality is high. Fulminant liver failure can be experimentally induced in mice by administering lipopolysaccharides (LPS) and galactosamine. Professor Masatoshi Yamazaki of Teikyo University's Department of Pharmacy investigated the liver protective effect of AHCC. Both galactosamine and LPS were administered simultaneously to mice pretreated with AHCC, and compared to mice that did not receive AHCC. In the group of mice that did not get AHCC, three out of the ten died within twenty-four hours. There were no deaths in the AHCC group. It was clear that AHCC demonstrated a protective effect on the liver, even in the extreme condition of fulminant liver failure induced by drugs.

AHCC is also effective against liver damage caused by cancer chemotherapy as well as chronic liver disease caused by alcohol abuse. The liver is always exposed to challenges in everyday life: medicines, alcohol, food additives, viruses, and the like. Because of its liver protective effect, AHCC can be used for health maintenance (Figure 3.3).

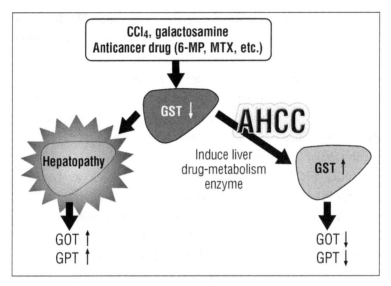

Figure 3.3 AHCC's liver protective activity

AHCC PREVENTS OPPORTUNISTIC INFECTION

Opportunistic infections are infections that occur with patients who have reduced immunity. In recent years the greatest problem with infections in hospitals is the often untreatable infection from methicillin-resistant *Staphylococcus aureus* (MRSA). Other types of opportunistic infections are candidiasis from *Candida albicans,* pseudomonas infections from *Pseudomonas aeruginosa* infection, and other infections, which are sometimes life-threatening. Opportunistic infections are difficult to treat with antibiotics alone. There is a demand for the development of medical treatments that can fortify compromised immunity.

Professor Shigeru Abe of the Research Center for Medical Mycology at Teikyo University experimented on mice and confirmed that AHCC was clearly effective in the prevention and treatment of opportunistic infections. Professor Abe created infection models by administering the anticancer drug cyclophosphamide in the peritoneal cavity of mice to lower their immunity and make them vulnerable to infection in advance. He then proceeded to infect them with various microbes in their condition of lowered immunity, in which their susceptibility to infections was high. Bacterial pathogens such as *Pseudomonas aeruginosa* and MRSA, and fungal pathogens like candida were used to infect the mice. In all cases of infection, there was at least an extension in the survival time and often a preventive effect when AHCC was administered (see Figure 3.4).

People with low immune competence, such as patients undergoing chemotherapy, have to be cautious about contracting infections. Elderly people are also at great risk. In people over the age of sixty-five, bronchitis can rapidly progress to a life-threatening pneumonia, which is a leading cause of death. Healthy elderly people can reduce this risk and improve their resistance by taking AHCC.

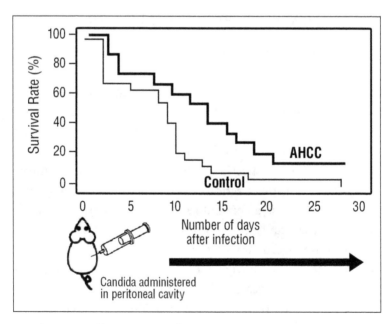

Figure 3.4 Life-extending effect of oral administration of AHCC in candida-infected mouse models

AHCC PREVENTS VIRAL INFECTIONS

AHCC has been shown to prevent various types of viral infections in animal models. AHCC increased the survival rate of young mice infected with the influenza virus. Mice treated with AHCC also lost less weight from the disease. Virus levels in the lung were reduced in the AHCC-treated group, and the lung tissue showed rapid signs of healing the mucous membranes. A study on the preventive potential of AHCC for avian flu was conducted at the College of Veterinary Medicine at the South China Agricultural University. Mice treated with AHCC were compared with untreated mice. AHCC significantly raised the survival rate, and even after reinfection with the virus on the twenty-first and twenty-eighth days after treatment, the survival rate stayed at 20–30 percent. Another study in which mice were infected with West Nile virus (WNV) showed similar results. Mice pretreated for seven days with AHCC had an increase in survival and a decreased viral load four days after infection.

AHCC PREVENTS INFECTION BY REDUCING THE EFFECTS OF STRESS

The relation between stress and immunity has been studied extensively with various types of stressors. Stress reliably lowers NK cell activity, among other effects. AHCC not only increases NK cell activity, but it also may have direct effects on reducing stress by lowering the levels of stress-related hormones. One unusual type of stress is experienced in spaceflight conditions. Researchers at Morehouse School of Medicine used a model called the Hindlimb Unloading Model that simulates spaceflight in mice. One of the effects of stress from spaceflight is impairment of the immune response and resistance to infection. Mice subjected to these conditions using this spaceflight simulation model were infected with the bacterium *Klebsiella pneumoniae,* a bacterium that causes pneumonia and other diseases. It is also often antibiotic-resistant. Klebsiella tends to occur in people with weakened immune systems or underlying chronic diseases, like an opportunistic infection. Once again, an untreated group of mice was compared to a group pretreated with AHCC. The mice pretreated with AHCC, followed by continued treatment with AHCC, had a much lower rate of death by Klebsiella infection than their untreated counterparts. Greater effects from AHCC were found in mice that had suppressed immunity. Mice treated with AHCC were protected to a greater extent than normally caged mice. This suggests that AHCC may be even more effective when the immune system is compromised.

ANTI-INFLAMMATORY EFFECT OF AHCC

Inflammation is a defensive reaction that attempts to eliminate the noxious stimulation of bacterial pathogens, and is a manifestation of the immune reaction. However, if this protective reaction is excessive or occurs unnecessarily, the body is harmed by the reaction. Many allergic disorders fall into this category: Atopic dermatitis, pollen allergy, and allergic asthma are the most common allergic disorders; autoimmune diseases, such as rheumatoid arthritis and collagen diseases like lupus (SLE: systemic lupus erythematosus), are also inflammatory immune system reactions, similar to allergic reactions that can result in tissue damage.

In general, steroidal and/or nonsteroidal anti-inflammatory drugs are used to treat these allergic disorders. These drugs are often ineffective and their side effects often cause harm. Dr. Satoshi Yui of Teikyo University's Department of Pharmacy observed the level of inflammation by measuring the peritoneal white cell count of mice in which inflammation was artificially induced. He found that the inflammation was contained in mice that were given an AHCC solution to drink, compared to

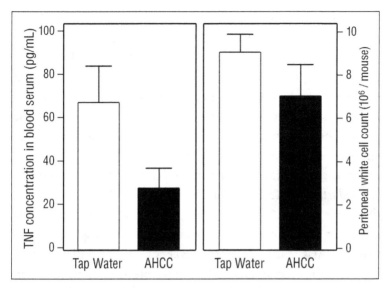

Figure 3.5 Effect of AHCC on blood serum TNF concentration and peritoneal cavity white cell count of mice with induced inflammation in the peritoneal cavity

mice that were given tap water only (see Figure 3.5). The concentration of the inflammatory cytokine TNF-α (tumor necrosis factor) in the serum was also reduced in the mice that were given AHCC. It was concluded that AHCC keeps inflammation under control.

AHCC IS A VERSATILE IMMUNOMODULATOR

An immunomodulator is a substance that alters, suppresses, or strengthens the immune system. AHCC has a much broader impact than conventional immunomodulators because it has a *normalizing* regulatory effect. This means that it stimulates immunity when there is an inhibited response, but also calms excessive immune reactions. The capability of AHCC to control excessive immune reactions was also confirmed in the above-referenced study on inflammation. A persuasive illustration is the effect of AHCC on cancer. One type of cytokine production stimulated by AHCC is TNF-α. As its name implies, tumor necrosis factor stimulates the breakdown of tumors. In a cancer condition, this is a valuable stimulus to the healing process. On the other hand, one of the goals of treatment in rheumatoid arthritis is to reduce or eliminate the presence of TNF-α, because it is a proinflammatory cytokine. We want its proinflammatory effect when there are tumors, but not when there is arthritis. In an arthritis condition, however, we see that AHCC stimulates the *reduction* of TNF-α. This normalizing effect seems to be the result of AHCC strengthening the function of the immune system in the function where it most needs strengthening and support. AHCC also decreased levels of another inflammatory marker, calprotectin. Like TNF-α, calprotectin counters cancer. In patients or test animals with cancer, calprotectin, like TNF-α, is increased, just as calprotectin levels are decreased when there is inflammation.

Dr. Mitsuaki Iwamoto of the Enzankai Medical Corporation in Sapporo, Japan, has reported cases of improved symptoms among rheumatoid arthritis patients who have taken AHCC continuously. Rheumatoid arthritis is known to be a chronic autoimmune inflammatory disease. Based on his observations, AHCC may also be used to treat symptoms of arthritis.

IMPLICATIONS OF THE EFFECTS OF AHCC ON THE INFLAMMATORY MECHANISM

Another marker of inflammation is C-reactive protein (CRP). Researchers at the National Cancer Institute in Bangkok, Thailand gave terminal liver cancer patients 3g a day of AHCC in a region of Thailand that has the highest rate of liver cancer in the world. After taking AHCC for six months, liver function levels in these patients returned to normal. In addition, the levels of CRP returned to normal, but they rose again if the AHCC dosage was stopped. C-reactive protein is high when there are infections, inflammatory bowel disease, pancreatitis, and certain cancers. There is a strong relationship between circulating CRP and cardiovascular disease. Blood levels of CRP are an indication of increased danger of heart attacks and strokes. AHCC has demonstrated its ability to reduce inflammation and also to reduce high levels of CRP. It is possible that the anti-inflammatory properties of AHCC can be used to prevent cardiovascular disease.

Several studies have shown that AHCC can increase nitric oxide production. In the case of cardiovascular disease, nitric oxide production has significant benefits. Nitric oxide protects the blood vessels' smooth muscle tissue from harmful constriction. This permits the flexibility needed for blood to circulate at lower pressure. It regulates platelet function and prevents the formation of dangerous clots. Nitric oxide also reduces arterial plaque. As an antioxidant, it calms the underlying inflammation that causes plaque to deposit. Nitric oxide also lowers cholesterol through its antioxidant activity. This is another mechanism by which AHCC could prevent cardiovascular disease.

AHCC increases levels of an anti-inflammatory hormone called leptin. In addition to its anti-inflammatory activity, leptin also plays a key role in fat metabolism and appetite regulation. These preliminary experimental trials show that AHCC holds promise for treating inflammatory diseases, cardiovascular protection, and even for weight control.

RESEARCH ON THE ANTIOXIDANT PROPERTIES OF AHCC

Oxidants in the environment and foods, environmental toxins, and anticancer drugs all increase the activity of oxygen in our bodies. Stress on our minds and bodies also increases this process of oxidation. Tissue cells and blood cells get damaged in a body with increased oxidation. This is an important factor in the aging process and in various diseases like cancer and lifestyle-related diseases like diabetes and heart disease.

Professor Shigeru Matsuzaki of the Dokkyo University School of Medicine's Biochemistry Department studied the antioxidant effect of AHCC by examining what kind of effect AHCC has on the active oxygen that is generated by anticancer drugs. Professor Matsuzaki's experiment is described below.

Apoptosis of thymus cells (tissues necessary for early-stage immunity development) that caused the fragmentation of the DNA of the thymus cells was seen in a group of rats that were administered the adrenal cortical hormone (steroid) dexamethasone. The thymus is the location where the T cells mature. Fragmentation of DNA was not observed in rats that were treated with AHCC in advance, and the apoptosis (cell death) of thymus cells was also controlled. Since dexamethasone causes damage to organs by generating active oxygen, the antioxidant activity of AHCC was thought to be responsible for protecting the thymus from damage. We should also look at the potential of AHCC to recover the immunity that is lowered by the use of steroids.

AHCC also demonstrated a protective effect in the case of damage by ferric nitrilotriacetate (FNT), another powerful oxidant. A marker substance in the urine that indicates DNA damage (8-OH-dG) was elevated after administering FNT to rats. There was no rise in this marker in FNT-treated rats after administering AHCC. Liver damage markers in the blood—GOT and GPT, and CPK (creatine phosphokinase) a marker of disordered muscle activity—also increased on administering FNT, but the liver function markers were maintained at normal values when AHCC was used. The lipid peroxides, products of damaging oxidation, and CPK activity were also maintained near the normal values.

Based on these results, Professor Matsuzaki came to the conclusion that AHCC reduces carcinogenesis and organ damage caused by DNA degradation and suppression of biomembrane oxidation. He was unable to conclude whether AHCC itself is effective or whether the enzymes with antioxidant effects in the body are stimulated by taking AHCC. Professor Matsuzaki pointed out that AHCC has demonstrated the capability to induce enzymes that eliminate active oxygen like superoxide dismutase (SOD). (See Figure 3.6.)

Oxidation means the deterioration or aging of tissue cells. The aging of tissue cells comes in the form of various diseases. AHCC, which demonstrates an antioxidant effect, holds the promise of being effective in the prevention and treatment of many chronic diseases, including cancer.

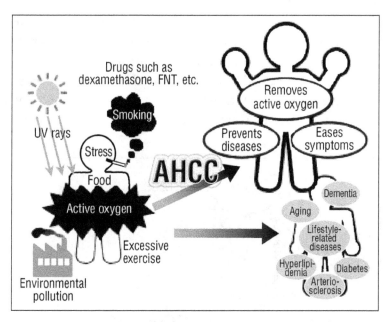

Figure 3.6 Antioxidative effect of AHCC

AHCC REDUCES STRESS AND BALANCES MIND AND BODY

The endocrine, immune, and nervous systems all interact with one another to maintain balance in our body. When there is stress on the nervous system, it affects the endocrine and immune systems and disrupts this balance, which can result in physical ailments and diseases. When our body undergoes stress, the hypothalamus sends signals to the adrenal cortex. An elevation in the secretion of the hormone corticosterone occurs. Corticosterone causes atrophy of organs related to immunity, like the thymus and the lungs; decreases the number of immune cells; and decreases the production of various cytokines, all of which leads to reduced immune competence (Figure 3.7).

Professor Shigeru Matsuzaki of Dokkyo University School of Medicine inflicted confinement stress on rats that were administered AHCC in advance and on rats that did not receive AHCC (the rats were tied up and immersed in water). Although the rats' blood sugar levels increased, due to the rise in secretion of adrenalin caused by acute stress in the untreated rats, there was hardly any increase in the blood sugar levels in rats under stress that received AHCC. Even the level of adrenalin secretion was controlled in the AHCC-treated rats. It can be seen from these

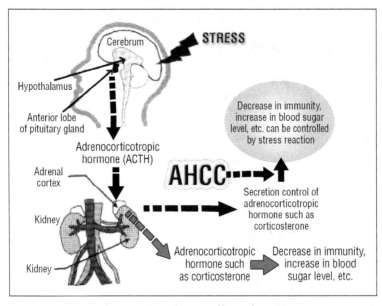

Figure 3.7 Antistress effect of AHCC

results that AHCC alleviates stress and contributes to maintaining the balance of mind and body. In this context we might say that AHCC is a nutrient, a food, that regulates the balance of immunity, the nervous response to stress, and the endocrine system. This stress-reducing property is important in preventing and treating most diseases.

THE USE OF AHCC IN VETERINARY HOSPITALS

In recent years there have been reports of lifestyle-related diseases and malignant diseases in dogs and cats. Malignant diseases and reduction in the quality of life (QOL), especially in aged dogs and cats, have become a serious problem for pet owners. Assistant Professor Masato Kuwahara of Nihon University's Department of Veterinary Radiation Research and a veterinarian by the name of Takahashi of the AHCC/Better Shark Research Association examined the effect of AHCC and shark cartilage on breast cancer tumors in dogs. AHCC (50mg/kg), used as an immune stimulant, and shark cartilage (100mg/kg), used as an angiogenesis inhibitor, were given twice a day with food to sixty-two dogs. Angiogenesis inhibitors prevent formation of blood vessels and therefore starve tumors by depriving them of blood vessels to bring nutrients for their survival. The protocol was given to the sixty-two dogs with breast tumors for over sixty days and the results were analyzed. The combination was found to have an antitumor effect in twenty-nine cases (46.8 percent) and to improve QOL in forty-five cases (72.6 percent).

The breakdown of the twenty-nine cases with the antitumor effect was as follows: very effective—six cases (9.78 percent); effective—twenty-three cases (37.1 percent). Tumor progression was halted in a total of twenty-four cases (38.7 percent) (see Figure 3.8).

As shown in Figure 3.9, the effect on QOL was as follows: Out of the sixty-two cases, there was an improvement in forty-five cases (72.6 percent) and no change in seventeen cases (27.4 percent). Further progression of the disease was not found in any of the cases.

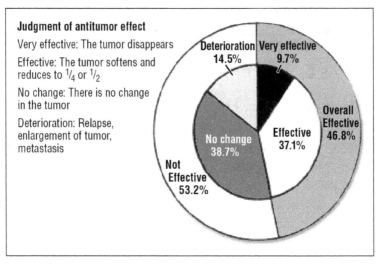

Figure 3.8 Effect of AHCC + shark cartilage on breast tumors in dogs

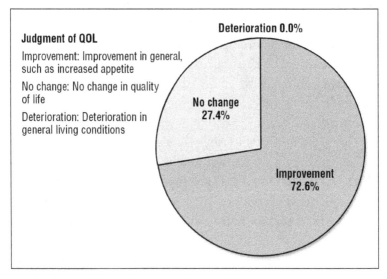

Figure 3.9 Effect of AHCC + shark cartilage with regard to QOL

In 1996 in Yokohama Dr. Toshihiko Okamoto, a veterinarian, removed a mixed tumor of flat epithelial cancer and fibrous sarcoma in the nasal cavity of a medium-sized dog (male, nine years old) and thereafter prescribed concomitant use of AHCC and shark cartilage with anticancer drugs. It was necessary to repeat the operation several times, but six years later there was hardly any tumor in the nasal region and the dog's QOL was reported to be excellent.

Another veterinarian, Dr. Mizobuchi of Takamatsu City removed a malignant breast tumor from a dog (female, three years old) and prescribed AHCC twice a day. He reported that there was no recurrence of cancer, even after one year. This became his standard treatment for breast cancer cases and in all cases the results have been excellent. There have been no side effects in any of the cases, and improved QOL and improved appetite have been observed, even in terminal cases.

Another veterinarian, Dr. Miura of Amagasaki City, uses AHCC as a postoperative cancer treatment. He removed a mammary adenoma (a benign tumor of glandular origin) from a small dog (female, eight years old) in 1999. The dog was given AHCC for over three years and has had no recurrence of the tumor. The dog remains in very good health.

Many veterinarians have confirmed that if it is possible to give animals AHCC, beneficial changes definitely appear within a few weeks, and even weak animals get a new lease on life. There are even reports that AHCC is effective against various age-related diseases, such as reduction of cataracts in old dogs.

CHAPTER 4

AHCC and Clinical Trials

The Helsinki Declaration, adopted by the World Medical Association in 1964 in Finland, is a Declaration of Human Rights based on the Nuremberg Code, established in 1947. It was specifically stated in this declaration that the well-being of human test subjects takes priority over scientific and social benefits in any clinical trials (Helsinki Declaration; Basic principles, Articles 1-6). In other words, injuring the life or health of a test subject in the name of science or development of medicines is prohibited, even if it is for research that holds promise of achieving significant scientific and social advances. Today it is still valued worldwide as the ethical and scientific standard for medical research. The standards for clinical trials are given more specifically in GCP (Good Clinical Practice = Practice standards of clinical trials of medicines), based on the intent of the Helsinki Declaration.

There are three stages (called phases) in clinical trials, as described below. Development of medications is carried out to confirm the safety and efficiency in each phase in an ethical manner. The results of each test implemented as a clinical trial are reviewed independently by ethics committees that uphold community standards.

Phase 1: In a small group of healthy adult volunteers, the candidate substance to be tested is first administered at a very low dose. The dosage is increased step-by-step and is periodically checked for safety.

Phase 2: When the candidate substance shows an effect, its safety, efficacy, and usage (dose, method of administration, etc.) are tested on a comparatively small group of patients.

Phase 3: Efficacy, safety, and usage of the drug are then confirmed on a large number of patients.

Phase 1 clinical trials have recently been conducted with AHCC conforming to GCP standards. However, informed consent based on the spirit of the Helsinki Declaration has always been enforced when AHCC is used for research purposes: Patients were given complete information about AHCC "as a health food" and their consent was obtained. Until now, AHCC has been used in a total of around six hundred hospital facilities in Japan. All studies and tests have been carried out with special priority given to the well-being and safety of all patients.

To further underscore the safety issue, the mushrooms used to manufacture AHCC are ones that have been used as food since ancient times; their safety as food has been confirmed by long historical tradition. Moreover, AHCC itself has been used by hundreds of thousands of people for over fifteen years, and no severe side effects have been reported at the appropriate level of intake.

Informed consent refers to obtaining consent, or agreement, from a patient after giving sufficient explanation of the condition of the disease, the course of treatment, and the drugs to be administered. Informed consent is only obtained after ensuring that the patient has understood the explanation completely. If patients do not have a full grasp of the protocol, they would not be able to give their informed consent. So patients must listen carefully to the doctor's explanation, ask questions, and make sure they fully understand the implications of the proposed course of treatment.

REPORTS OF USAGE OF AHCC GATHERED FROM DOCTORS

Fundamental research and clinical studies into AHCC's safety and efficacy are being carried out vigorously in over six hundred medical institutions and in more than thirty universities in several countries. The results have been published by the AHCC Research Association, have been presented at many domestic and foreign conferences, and have appeared in numerous scientific journals. The expectations of AHCC and trust in its use are increasing day by day, especially in the field of cancer. In particular, groups within Japan, such as Hokkaido University Genetic Disease Research Institute, Teikyo University Department of Pharmacology, and Kansai Medical University Department of Medicine, are conducting ongoing research in this field.

PHASE 1 TRIALS FOR AHCC IN THE UNITED STATES

AHCC was tested with healthy volunteers in a recent study conducted by a team of researchers from Harvard, Yale, and the Amino Up Chemical Company in Japan. A group of volunteers were given a higher-than-normal dose of the supplement in liquid form. A small number of the subjects experienced temporary stomach discomfort and headache, but these effects were mild and lasted only a short time. There were no abnormalities found in any of the subjects, according to blood tests.

PHASE 2 TRIALS FOR AHCC IN THE UNITED STATES

Researchers in Japan worked with medical researchers at Yale University and confirmed that AHCC enhances immune function in a way that can prevent cancer in elderly people. The research showed that the immune-boosting and cancer-preventive cytokines IFN and TNF increased within four weeks of taking the recommended dose of AHCC. This immune-enhancing effect also persisted for at least a month after stopping the daily dose.

Another research study showed that AHCC is unlikely to cause increased toxicity when combined with chemotherapy or supportive therapies, such as antidepressants and antinausea medications.

A team of researchers at the M.D. Anderson Cancer Center of the University of Texas and Amino Up Chemical Company in Japan studied liver enzymes (the cytochrome P-450 family of enzymes) in an important liver detoxification pathway involved in drug metabolism. This is a pathway through which many chemotherapy drugs are metabolized. The results showed that AHCC is unlikely to cause increased toxicity when combined with chemotherapy or supportive therapies. Since AHCC does increase the activity of the cytochrome P-450 detoxification pathway, further investigation will be needed to see if there is any interaction between AHCC and any type of drug that uses this pathway.

AHCC IMPROVED FIVE-YEAR SURVIVAL RATES

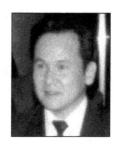

Dr. Yusai Kawaguchi of the Kansai Medical University Department of Surgery performed a clinical study that convincingly showed that the use of AHCC could remarkably enhance the five-year survival rate. He treated 132 stomach cancer patients with AHCC after surgery. Patients at stages I–IV were given 3g a day of AHCC and patients at stage IV were treated with 6g a day. Patients at stage II and higher were also given low-dose chemotherapy. In addition, he treated 113 patients with colon cancer. Patients at the early stages were treated with 3g of AHCC per day and patients at stages III and IV were given 6g a day in divided doses. Patients at stage II and higher were also given low-dose chemotherapy. An analysis of survival rates revealed that the five-year survival rates were remarkably enhanced.

AHCC INCREASES SURVIVAL TIME IN LATE-STAGE CANCER PATIENTS

Any treatment that can help late-stage cancer patients is worth its weight in gold. Researchers at the Faculty of Allied Health Sciences, Thammasat University, Rangsit Campus, Patumthani, Thailand, studied the use of AHCC with liver cancer patients at advanced stages. Forty-four patients were randomized and divided into an AHCC group, taking 6g a day, and a control group taking a placebo. In this study, AHCC clearly significantly increased survival time. In the study, the median patient survival time was twice as high in the AHCC group as in the control group. The results not only suggested that AHCC increased the probability of longer-term survival, but other factors the researchers monitored indicated that it also improved quality of life.

LIFE-EXTENDING EFFECT OF AHCC ON LIVER CANCER PATIENTS

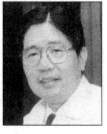

Since 1994 Professor Yasuo Kamiyama, chief of surgery at Kansai Medical University, has prescribed 3–6g of AHCC per day to hundreds of cancer patients, dividing it into three doses, and has observed the effects for over a decade. Most of these patients were liver cancer patients diagnosed with chronic hepatitis or cirrhosis, or both. This study has helped attract significant scientific and professional recognition to AHCC internationally, including an article published in 2002 in the prestigious *Journal of Hepatology*, a well-respected, peer-reviewed journal. The research was of exceptionally high quality, and has been carried out over an extended period with significant follow-up and monitoring of large numbers of cancer patients.

This procedure was then carried out on other cancer patients and the collective results were reported to the European Surgical Academy.

Objective

To administer AHCC to people who requested it after under-going liver resection surgery and being histologically diagnosed with hepatocellular carcinoma (HCC) between February 1992 and December 2000 in the Primary Surgery Department of Kansai Medical School.

Methodology & Outcome

AHCC-administered group: 107 patients (3g/day)

Group receiving no AHCC: 101 patients (control group)

The results of detailed statistical analysis carried out after the tests showed that the survival rate of the AHCC-administered group was significantly higher that the survival rate of the group who received no AHCC (see Figure 4.1).

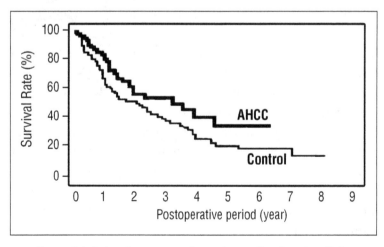

Figure 4.1 Rate of recurrence in post-resection hepatocellular carcinoma patients taking AHCC

TABLE 4.1 CANCER AND TUMOR MARKERS

CANCER	TUMOR MARKER
Lung cancer	CEA, CYFRA, NSE, ProGRP
Thyroid gland cancer	CEA, Calcitonin, Cycloglobulin
Esophageal cancer	SCC, CEA
Gastric cancer	CEA, CA 19-9
Colon cancer, Rectal cancer	CEA, CA 19-9
Liver cancer	AFP, PIVKA-1
Pancreatic cancer	CA 19-9, CA50; Elastase
Breast cancer	CEA, CA15-3
Gallbladder cancer, Bile duct cancer	CA19-9, CEA
Ovarian cancer	CA 125, STN
Cervical cancer	SCC
Prostate cancer	PSA, PAP, g-Sm
Urinary bladder cancer	BFP
Testicular cancer	AFP, Ak-P, hCG
Choriocarcinoma	hCG
Multiple myeloma	M protein, Bence-Jones protein

A follow-up survey was conducted for five years after the surgery for ten parameters to study the changes in the serological test data related to liver function. The results showed that there was a significant improvement in three parameters (AST, γGTP, and cholinesterase) in the AHCC-administered group.

Conclusion

These results suggest the possibility that intake of AHCC after HCC surgery may lead to improvement in hepatitis, prevention of relapse, and improvement in the survival rate.

> The five-year survival rate is the percentage of patients from the population of a certain kind of cancer who survive for five years from the first detection of cancer. Although it also depends on the type of cancer, patients are usually considered "cured" if there is no metastasis or relapse over a period of five years.

In an overall impression of this report, Professor Kamiyama identified the possibility of a decrease in hepatitis virus and a suppression of the liver cirrhosis caused by chronic hepatitis. When 6g of AHCC per day were administered orally in patients with a large amount of fluid from ascites and an increase in the level of tumor markers associated with HCC, four cases were reported in which a decrease in the peritoneal fluid, a decrease in the bilirubin levels, and a decrease in the tumor markers (PIVKA-H) were seen. It is believed that AHCC can be used as a symptomatic treatment for ascites, which does not respond well to most types of diuretic drugs, albumin drugs, or drainage.

> A tumor marker is a substance that indicates the presence of certain types of cancer cells. Tumor markers can also be defined as substances produced by cancer cells, or substances produced by normal cells in response to the presence of cancer cells, which can be used for diagnosis and evaluation of treatment progress (see Table 4.1, "Cancer and Tumor Markers").

USE OF AHCC IN THE TERMINAL STAGES OF CANCER

A group of doctors led by Dr. Katsuaki Uno, managing director of Comfort Hospital, Yokohama, set up the tumor immunity Outpatient Department in the same hospital. They observed the effect of AHCC in cancer treatment by targeting 195 patients who had checkups between June 1998 and November 2000.

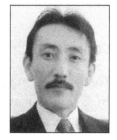

All of the 195 cancer patients were diagnosed as stage IV patients considered to have a poor survival prognosis and not treatable. The study was limited to patients who had not undergone treatment with surgery, chemotherapy, or radiation within one month of being enrolled in the study.

Patients with stage IV cancer are those with no hope of response to treatment. The doctor has given up hope that conventional treatment can effect any substantive, positive change. The summary of the report by Dr. Uno is as follows:

Subjects

A total of 195 patients with gastric cancer, colon cancer, liver cell cancer, pancreatic cancer, lung cancer, breast cancer, and ovarian cancer who satisfied the above-mentioned conditions.

Methodology & Outcome

Six grams of AHCC per day were given continuously for six months. Other suitable immune stimulants were given along with it. The immunological tests that were carried out during this period included natural killer (NK) cell activation and Th1-related cytokine (IFN-γ, IL-12) production. There were thirty-six cases whose immunological parameter evaluation was made in the second month, twenty-six cases in the fourth month, and eighteen cases in the sixth month. Two cases of deaths caused by progression of the cancer were reported; no cause-and-effect relationship with the intake of AHCC was identified.

A significant rise was seen in NK cell activity, and IFN-γ and IL-12 production, within six months of starting to take AHCC.

Immunotherapy patients who were given 6g/day of AHCC and who fulfilled the following conditions were studied:

- Measurement of immunological parameters before and after starting the treatment (2 months)

- Patients whose efficacy rate could be judged for 6 months after starting the treatment.

The PS evaluation (evaluation of the functioning capability of cancer patients) before and after completion of the test was compared, and it was found that there was a significant increase in functioning capability after taking AHCC compared to before taking AHCC. The efficacy rate was Complete Response (CR): 17 cases; Partial Response (PR): 97 cases; No Change (NC): 27 cases; and Progression of Disease (PD): 54 cases (see Table 4.2).

	COMPLETE RESPONSE	PARTIAL RESPONSE	NO CHANGE	PROGRESSION OF DISEASE	TOTAL
TABLE 4.2 AHCC IMMUNOTHERAPY AND EFFICACY RATE					
Number of patients	17	97	27	54	195
Percentage	8.8	49.7	13.8	27.7	100.0

After administering AHCC to these stage IV cancer patients, researchers began to approach cancer treatment as an effort to activate the entire immune mechanism. They saw improvement in the activity of the NK cells, which are a type of cancer-destroying white cell, increasing the production of interleukin-12 (IL-12), and inducing the production of cytokines, such as interferon (IFN-γ). Dr. Uno reported a total of 114 cases of complete recovery (CR) and partial improvement (PR). There were 27 cases in which the cancer progress had been stopped (NC) in six months after the commencement of the intake of AHCC. This result is remarkable, considering that all of the test subjects were at the terminal stage of cancer.

The cancer treatment efficacy rate is generally judged at the following levels:

CR (Complete Response) = Tumor disappeared in less than 4 weeks

PR (Partial Response) = Tumor shrank to 50 percent in less than 4 weeks from the beginning of the treatment

NC (No change) = No change was seen

PD (Progression of Disease) = Growth of the tumor and progression of disease

THE USE OF AHCC FOR BRAIN CANCER

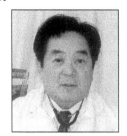

Researcher: Dr. Myousei Shimizu,
   Shibutami Central Hospital (Iwate
   Prefecture)
Subject: Male, 21 years old
Diagnosis: Primary brain tumor
   (medulloblastoma)

Dizziness, narrowing of the visual field, and staggering were observed from the beginning, and thereafter the patient experienced headaches, queasiness, nausea, loss of appetite, and an inability to walk. He consulted a teaching hospital, and was diagnosed with medulloblastoma. He was hospitalized on the recommendation of the doctor. At that time, the doctor noted the following:

> Medulloblastoma is a type of brain tumor that permeates the interior of the brain. There is no clear demarcation between tumor cells and healthy brain cells. Since there are tumor cells and healthy brain cells in close proximity, it is impossible to remove the tumor completely. The disease has already progressed to the terminal stage. Even if we treat it with radiation therapy and anticancer drugs, his survival time is estimated at six months or less.

Doctors started the treatment with anticancer drugs and cerebrospinal pressure was reduced instantly. Later, radiation was carried out. The doctors recommended that "It would be better if he spent time at home with his family as long as he is on his feet," due to his low chance of recovery and his limited expected survival time. He was then discharged from the hospital. After leaving the hospital, he started AHCC and other immunotherapies. The tumor disappeared within four months. Furthermore, hardly any symptoms were seen after a few months and he was able to get on with his routine college life. Three years later, during a routine medical checkup at the hospital, he was diagnosed as "completely cured" after multiple diagnostic tests, including an MRI.

Researcher: Dr. Myousei Shimizu, Shibutami Central Hospital
(Iwate Prefecture)
Subject: Female, 64 years old
Diagnosis: Brain tumor (brain stem tumor)

The patient had headaches, dizziness, nausea, and persistent pain in the back of the head. She consulted a neurosurgeon at a prefectural hospital and was diagnosed with a brain tumor. As the tumor was on the brain stem, an area that cannot be operated on, she was told that "Treatment is not possible and [she] could die at any time." After that, she immediately consulted Shibutami Central Hospital. From that day she took AHCC and other immunotherapies. After three months the tumor had shrunk by half and had completely disappeared after eleven months! She reported that her "physical condition was good and the headaches have also gone. I can move around energetically every day."

Researcher: Dr. Francisco Contreras,
Oasis Hospital (Mexico)
Subject: Female, 33 years old
Diagnosis: Metastatic brain tumor
(primary focus: breast cancer, lung cancer, brain metastasis)

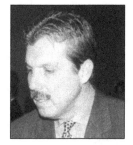

This patient started taking AHCC along with anticancer drugs when brain metastasis was confirmed. The metastasis disappeared two months later. Though the disappearance of the metastasis was assumed to be the direct effect of the anticancer drugs, the patient continued to take AHCC. Her immunity was immensely increased and recurrence of the tumor was not seen. Although treatment with anticancer drugs failed in the case of metastasis in the bones and lungs over time, the metastasis was reduced by the intake of AHCC and an excellent prognosis was envisioned.

Alternative treatments are researched in this hospital and although the emphasis is on diet therapy and palliative care, AHCC along with anticancer drugs were given to eighteen patients at a terminal stage of cancer. More than 80 percent of the patients showed an improvement in their subjective symptoms (quality of life—QOL). In the blood test results, we observed that the number of white blood cells (especially neutrophils), red blood cells, and platelets had increased by 50 percent (see Figure 4.2)

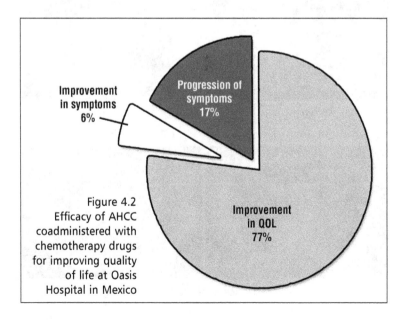

Improvement in symptoms 6%

Progression of symptoms 17%

Improvement in QOL 77%

Figure 4.2
Efficacy of AHCC coadministered with chemotherapy drugs for improving quality of life at Oasis Hospital in Mexico

THE USE OF AHCC IN LUNG CANCER

Researcher: Dr. Katsuaki Uno, Comfort Hospital (Yokohama)
Subject: Male, 70 years old
Diagnosis: Lung cancer

This patient had a history of myocardial infarction, so surgery was considered ill-advised. A large tumor was clearly seen in the CT scans of the patient before starting AHCC and other immunotherapies (Figure 4.3). The CT scans taken immediately after AHCC had been started showed that there was an increase in the size of the tumor, instead of a reduction. However, recovery/enhancement of immune strength was confirmed in the test values of the cancer immunity screening since taking AHCC. In the CT scans taken two months later, it was observed that the tumor had shrunk in size. In the CT scan taken after eight months, the tumor had shrunk to the point where it had almost disappeared.

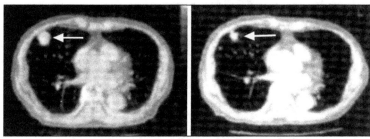

1. Original CT scan	3. CT scan two months later
2. Scan right after starting AHCC	4. CT scan eight months later

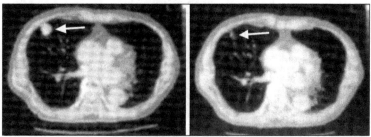

Figure 4.3 CT scans of the patient's lungs

Researcher: Dr. Yasunari Fujioka, Fujioka
  Clinic (Kumamoto)
Subject: Male, 65 years old
Diagnosis: Lung cancer

The patient consulted this hospital after he noticed a lump on the right side of his neck. Lung cancer and lymph node metastases in the right neck region were diagnosed and he was asked to undergo a thorough medical checkup in an institute for specialized treatment. As it was already too late for an operation, chemotherapy with anticancer drugs was suggested, but the patient refused the drugs because of their side effects. He consulted this hospital again and AHCC was started a month later. His general condition was good, except for a hoarse voice. No change in the size of the tumor was recognized from the time of diagnosis in the CT scans of the chest (see Figure 4.4, top) taken four months after starting treatment.

Although an increase in the size of the tumor was recognized in the CT scan of the chest taken three months later (center), there was no notable change in the patient's overall condition. There was no change in the tumor size in the CT scans taken four months after that (bottom), compared to those taken previously. The patient contin-

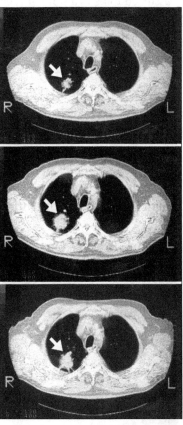

Figure 4.4 CT scans of the chest

ued visiting this hospital as an outpatient. Though he was living with cancer, other than the hoarseness of his voice, no symptoms (such as cough, productive cough, chest pain, or dyspnea) were seen, and there was no proliferation of the tumor.

If we study this case thoroughly, we could say that AHCC had an equal or greater cancer-controlling effect than the anticancer drugs. Moreover, there was no fear of side effects, as seen in anticancer drugs. AHCC made a huge contribution to the QOL of the patient.

When development of cancer is stopped by immunotherapy, it is assumed to be in a state of coexistence with cancer. This is a very good condition for the patient, since the cancer is in a dormant state and future treatment can be postponed if this condition is maintained.

CASES OF USE OF AHCC FOR CANCER OF THE DIGESTIVE SYSTEM

Researcher: Dr. Yusai Kawaguchi, Primary Surgery, Kansai Medical University (Osaka)
Diagnosis: Cancer of the entire digestive system

Methodology & Outcome

The treatment policy of this department is to perform surgery first, followed by low-dose chemotherapy, then radiation treatment, and finally AHCC. Dr. Kawaguchi and his team collected data on patients who were operated on for various types of digestive system cancers and given AHCC over the five-year period from April 1995 through 2000. Patients who were given chemotherapy were also included in this data.

There were ninety-four cases of stomach cancer. The survival rate from stage IIa to stage IIIa among these cases was 100 percent with no relapse or metastasis, even at stage III. There was only one case of liver metastasis in a patient at stage IIIa. Even two years after the start of AHCC treatment, there was only one case of relapse at stage IIIb, but with no metastasis. In one case of stage III, there was no relapse or metastasis seen even two years after the start of treatment with AHCC.

There were eighty-two cases of patients taking AHCC after colon cancer surgery. The five-year survival rate up to stage IIIa was 100 percent and metastasis was reported in only two cases at stage IIIa. Relapse and metastasis were seen in about half the cases at stage IIIb. In two cases of stage III, both showed liver metastasis and lung metastases.

TNM Classification

When the stage of cancer is clarified, we sometimes get a description like "T0N1M0." This is determined by three factors: the size of the tumor, the degree of metastasis in the peripheral lymph nodes, and the presence of metastasis in remote internal organs. This is called the TNM classification and is used as an international code. This classification is carried out by combining these three factors: T = Tumor, N = Node (lymph node), and M = Metastasis (see Table 4.3).

Stage classifications are based on the TNM classification system and are used to demarcate the rate of progression of the cancer and its degree of proliferation. Since this classification is based on clinical studies, it is called Clinical Development Stage Classification. It is normally divided into four stages, from an early stage (stage I) to the terminal stage (stage IV). Moreover, there are subdivisions marked by the letters a and b at each stage. Stage classifications are determined by the condition of internal organs similar to the TNM classification (see Table 4.4).

TABLE 4.3 TNM (TUMOR-NODE-METASTASIS) CLASSIFICATION

FACTOR	DEGREE	DEFINITION
Primary tumor	T0	No tumor (there is no hardening)
T: tumor	T1–T4	Depends on tumor size and degree of penetration, classified according to which organ is affected.
Lymph node metastasis	N0	No lymph node metastasis
N: Lymph nodes	N1–N4	Classified according to the degree of lymph node metastasis from the affected organ.
Remote organ metastasis	M0	No metastasis is seen in remote organs
M: Metastasis	M1	Metastasis to remote organs

TABLE 4.4 STAGE CLASSIFICATION OF UTERINE CANCER

STAGE	DEFINITION
0 stage	Cancer cells are confined to the epithelium
Ia stage	Cancer cells penetrate beyond the basal membrane of the epithelium, but within 5mm
Ib stage	Penetration is beyond 5mm, but has only reached the cervical region
IIa stage	Penetration has gone beyond the cervical region, but cancer cells have not penetrated beyond one-third of the vaginal wall
IIb stage	Cancer cells have penetrated the tissue that supports the uterus at the bottom of the pelvis
IIIa stage	Cancer cells have penetrated beyond one-third of the vagina wall
IIIb stage	Cancer cells have penetrated to all points of the pelvic wall
IVa stage	Cancer cells have penetrated to the mucous membrane of the urinary bladder or rectum
IVb stage	The penetration of cancer cells has spread beyond the pelvic wall and metastasis is seen in remote organs, such as the lungs and the liver

Low-dose chemotherapy and AHCC were started in another patient with metastasis in both lungs one year after rectal cancer surgery during the stage when metastasis was observed. Even though the area of metastasis of this patient slowly enlarged, instead of receding, the patient's physical condition was good and he visited the hospital for regular checkups.

Liver metastasis appeared in a patient one year after surgery for sigmoid colon cancer. The right lobe of the liver was excised and chemotherapy, together with AHCC, was soon initiated. After one year there was still no relapse or metastasis.

Another patient underwent total removal of the stomach after detection of stomach cancer, followed by removal of the gallbladder, partial removal of the small intestine, removal of the left adrenal gland, and partial excision of the peritoneum due to extensive metastasis. This patient was at stage III and had an estimated survival time of three to six months. Survival time was actually two years after the operation with the use of anticancer drugs and AHCC. A relevant tumor marker (CEA) also stayed in the normal range.

Based on this, it is believed that AHCC is useful in the prevention of relapse and metastasis of gastrointestinal-tract cancers, and for improving the QOL when relapse or metastasis does occur. This life-extension effect can also be expected when cancer is considered to be at a terminal stage.

Researcher: Dr. Tomoyasu Sakurai, Sakurai Gastroenterological Clinic (Sapporo)
Subject: Male, 54 years old
Diagnosis: Liver cancer

This patient had various symptoms, such as mild fever, headaches, and a cold in May 1999. Another hospital diagnosed liver hypertrophy. Tests performed after hospitalization led to a diagnosis of liver cancer with cirrhosis, caused by hepatitis C. He was told that he had approximately six months left to live. He was given anticancer drugs intravenously and a transcatheter arterial embolization (TAE) in the liver. TAE is carried out in patients who have had surgery for liver cancer. It is a treatment in which a catheter is inserted into an artery in the liver by the same method used in angiography, and a substance that packs the blood vessels (embolus substance) is injected through the catheter. When the arterial blood is cut off by this method, liver cancer cells cannot survive, since their only source of blood is from the artery.

The patient consulted this hospital, hoping to get supplemental alternative treatment. The observation of multiple liver cancers with liver cirrhosis was confirmed by an ultrasound of the abdomen. The doctor in charge decided to discharge him from the hospital on July 10 so he could spend as much time as possible with his family. He was then prescribed by this hospital AHCC and a traditional Chinese herbal formula, Ginseng and Dang Gui Ten, which consists of ten herbs for improving stamina and resistance.

He was advised to eat a healthy diet, get sufficient exercise, get sufficient sleep, and to maintain a cheerful and positive outlook to sustain his immunity. My own personal experience with colon cancer indicates that this kind of care of body and mind is very important for a positive outcome.

The patient was given dynamic injection treatment with anticancer drugs several times, and even though cirrhosis was clearly seen in the CT scan carried out a year later, no cancer was detected. The tumor marker AFP (alpha-fetoprotein) increased up to 40 but there was no change in this value beyond that. Two years later, there was no change from his previous condition and he continues with the dynamic injection treatment, AHCC, and traditional Chinese medicine. In this case, the result was obtained due to the combination of chemotherapy and supplemental alternative treatment.

Researcher: Dr. Katsuaki Uno, Comfort Hospital (Yokohama)
Subject: Male, 55 years old
Diagnosis: Cancer of esophageal flat epithelium

Methodology & Outcome

In this patient, esophageal cancer was diagnosed in a medical checkup. Surgery was recommended. The patient refused to undergo the operation because his elder brother had died after an operation for esophageal cancer. At his first visit to this hospital two months later, he was given the cancer immunity screening to determine his immune strength against cancer. Then he was started on immunotherapy, in which AHCC played the central role. There was clear improvement several months later in all the blood test values measured in the cancer immunity screening. The tumor in the esophagus had almost disappeared four months later. Figure 4.5 is an x-ray taken in October 1999, and it can be clearly seen that the esophagus is blocked by the tumor. Figure 4.6 is the x-ray taken in February 2000, in which can be seen that the tumor has clearly disappeared and the esophagus has returned to its original healthy state.

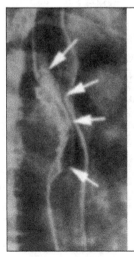

Figure 4.5
October 1999:
X-ray of
esophageal
tumor

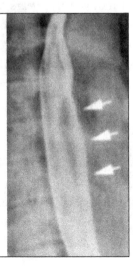

Figure 4.6
February 2000:
X-ray shows
tumor has
disappeared

Researcher: Professor Yasuo Kamiyama, Chief of Surgery,
  Kansai Medical University (Osaka)
Diagnosis: Pancreatic cancer

Methodology & Outcome

The incidence of pancreatic cancer increases every year; in the past twenty years the number of cases has increased by three to four times. Although the cause is not clearly known, it is assumed to be due to a growing incidence of poor eating habits, such as consuming a lot of foods high in animal fat or protein and an inadequate intake of vegetables.

Surgery is usually necessary, but in cases that are inoperable, treatments for pain, narrowing of the digestive tract, jaundice, and other symptoms are also necessary.

Survival time is typically short in most cases of pancreatic cancer treated at this hospital, and surgery is often impossible. In such cases, combined treatment of AHCC and other Western medicines are given. Four patients have survived for more than ten months and in one case, the patient's pancreatic cancer was confirmed by CT scan to have disappeared and the patient was still alive three years later. Improvement in QOL, such as pain relief, has also been observed.

It can't be stated conclusively that this effect of prolonging life is due to the intake of AHCC, because the patient sample size is too small, but it appears certain that the combined use of modern medicine and AHCC has reduced the pain of the patients.

Researcher: Dr. Yusai Kawaguchi, Primary Surgery, Kansai
  Medical University (Osaka)
Subject: Female, 65 years old
Diagnosis: Unresectable pancreatic cancer

Methodology & Outcome

When this patient was hospitalized in 2007, the tumor marker (CA 19-9 at 92.4 μ/ml; normal value is less than 37) had increased and it was a case in which surgery was not an option. Treatment with chemotherapy (5-FU and cisplatin), radiation therapy, and AHCC was started. It was found in the CT scan that the tumor was reduced in size after six months. After eight months, the tumor marker CA 19-9 had decreased remarkably to 12.6. There was no relapse or metastasis, and the patient continued to live healthily. In this case, combined use of low-dose chemotherapy and AHCC had been effective.

AHCC FOR GYNECOLOGICAL CANCERS

Researchers: Dr. Hiroshi Torishigeru, Fujimoto Hospital (Osaka) and Dr. Yusai Kawaguchi, Kansai Medical University (Osaka)
Diagnosis: Breast cancer, postsurgery

Methodology & Outcome

In a clinical study, 3g/day or 6g/day of AHCC was given as a post-operative supplemental treatment to twenty-nine patients who had undergone excision of breast cancer between January 1995 and September 1998. The survival rates obtained were studied by comparison to data (three-year postsurgical survival rate) of the Japan National Cancer Center. In studying the effects of AHCC, the following impressions were formed:

The survival rate was excellent (100 percent survival rate) in patients from stage I to stage III, and two in four cases of stage IV survived—a considerable life-extension effect. There are good chances of recovery from breast cancer if it is treated in the initial stages with excision or chemotherapy. Breast conservation surgery is widely used and stress on the patients is brought under control as much as possible. The role of AHCC in such cases is apparently to mitigate the side effects of the anticancer drugs and to prevent relapse or metastasis of the disease.

Researcher: Dr. Mototaka Oura, Oura
   Clinic (Osaka)
Subject: Female, 67 years old,
Diagnosis: Uterine cancer

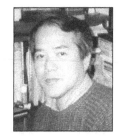

Methodology & Outcome

The patient underwent surgery for uterine cancer in a teaching hospital in June 2000. In the CT scan from July 2001, two metastatic lesions were found in the pelvis and the uterus was compressed, causing hydronephrosis. The patient underwent the operation for draining the urine and then consulted this hospital on July 27 for intense pain. She was advised to take 6g of AHCC, along with other health foods. At that time, she was in an inoperable condition and even refused radiation therapy. When she came to the hospital three months later, she was happy because the inflammation of the urinary tract had subsided, her fever had gone down, her physical condition was generally good, and she had gained weight. The next month a thorough checkup was carried out at the teaching hospital and the results revealed that the size of metastatic lesions had not changed, but the development of the cancer had apparently stopped. She was given nutritional guidance at that time and was told to change her diet to consist of mostly vegetables and fish. As of 2002, she was showing favorable progress and was living in a healthy condition.

This was an impressive case, since this patient was feeling rejuvenated, even though she suffered a relapse, metastasis, and various other complications after the operation. Her voice was strong and her laughter was free. Such a positive attitude greatly helps in the improvement of QOL.

Researcher: Dr. Susuma Konda, Uchinada
Onsen Hospital (Ishikawa)
Subject: Female, 84 years old
Diagnosis: Suspected uterine cancer

Methodology & Outcome

This patient complained of abdominal distention and loss of appetite in early September 1998. Ascites and edema were detected at the end of September. The tumor was not detected in the abdomen either by palpation or in diagnostic imaging, but the value of tumor marker CA125 was high (although tumor cells were not found in the peritoneal fluid). Ovarian or uterine cancer was suspected and a follow-up was carried out. She was further troubled by loss of appetite, edema, and ascites (fluid accumulation in the abdominal cavity). Her abdominal circumference had increased to approximately 90cm by the end of October. She started taking AHCC in December 1998 and soon recovered her appetite and a substantial decrease in edema was observed. The abdominal diameter was reduced to 73cm by February 1999. The CA125 level also returned to the normal range and she stopped taking AHCC in July of that year. In this patient the maximum value of CA125 had reached the extremely high value of 450 μ/m1. The normal range is less than 35 μ/ml. All other tumor markers showed normal values. This case was assumed to be a "false positive" disorder of CA125. Although endometriosis or pleural membrane or peritoneum disorders can be indicated in false positive disorders of CA125, this patient had a benign disorder of the peritoneum and, as such, blockage caused by arteriosclerosis of the mesenteric artery was conjectured. It has been observed that peritoneal fluid drains through the urine if AHCC is taken at the terminal stage of cancer. In this one situation, however, ascites from malignancy did not cause the increase in urine volume.

AHCC FOR BONE AND BLOOD CANCERS

Researcher: Dr. Myousei Shimizu, Shibutami Central Hospital (Iwate)
Subject: Female, 62 years old
Diagnosis: Multiple myeloma

Methodology & Outcome

This patient was diagnosed with multiple myeloma at the Japan National Cancer Center on April 18, 1999. She was already suffering from lumbar and midback pain, anemia, and a high fever. The doctor in charge explained that myeloma cells had proliferated in the spinal cord, and had damaged the vertebral body, causing osteoporosis. This led to a complex compression fracture of the spine, giving rise to lumbar and back pain. He also explained that he knew of no way that the pain could be alleviated because the penetration of the tumor cells had extended outside the vertebral body, compressing the nerves directly. So there was no known treatment. He suggested using Alkeran (an anticancer drug) and prednisone (a steroid), but explained that she had roughly six months left to live, at most. When AHCC and other immunotherapies were started, her physical condition improved gradually and eventually an apparent recovery was witnessed. About five months after starting the immunotherapy, a CT scan, an MRI, x-rays of the bones, and a bone marrow aspiration were conducted at the National Cancer Center. It was found that the cancer cells had disappeared. Blood tests also revealed that the patient was no longer anemic.

The patient was erroneously diagnosed with osteoporosis because of the pain in the lumbar region. This patient, diagnosed in October 2000 with stage IV multiple myeloma, improved remarkably with chemotherapy and AHCC. She was still alive as of March 2002, in good physical condition, and was maintaining a routine of normal activities.

Researcher: Dr. Tomoyasu Sakurai, Sakurai Gastroenterological Clinic (Sapporo)
Subject: Male, 32 years old
Diagnosis: Malignant lymphoma (non-Hodgkin's lymphoma, stage III)

Methodology & Outcome

In 1998 this patient was diagnosed with stage III malignant lymphoma and he consulted our clinic for a second opinion concerning his treatment. At that time, chemotherapy was recommended, and he was asked to undergo tests and treatment at a local hospital's Hematology Department. The doctor in charge explained that his relative prognosis was good and that because the patient was still young, recovery could be expected if the anti-cancer drug succeeded.

Instead of undergoing the recommended course of chemotherapy, the patient opted to come to this clinic for alternative treatment. He visited the hospital regularly and started the alternative treatment because, as he stated, "I want to carry out normal day-to-day activities and return to the office at any cost."

Along with AHCC and the Chinese herbal medicine Ginseng and Dang Gui Ten, he underwent psychotherapy. At each consultation he was told to be aware of his mental state and to try to stave off mental depression to keep up his immunity. He was asked to lead his everyday life positively and cheerfully, eat a balanced diet, exercise moderately, and get enough sleep. Though the doctors in the Department of Hematology at his local hospital did not imagine that the tumor would shrink with this alternative treatment, the cervical lymph nodes of both sides, which were palpable, and the auxiliary lymph nodes had shrunk within six months from the start of the treatment. His CT scans also revealed that the lymph nodes in the chest and abdomen had shrunk.

Reduction in the diameter of the lymph nodes from the thighs was seen in around the eighth month and the swelling of all the peripheral lymph nodes had disappeared by the third year after the start of the treatment. The exception was the lymph nodes above the clavicle, which were slightly enlarged. No swelling of the abdominal lymph nodes was observed in the ultrasound and the tumor had completely clinically disappeared when this patient visited the hospital as an outpatient in January 2002. This time he was able to perform all normal activities.

Researcher: Dr. Tomoyasu Sakurai, Sakurai Gastroenterological Clinic (Sapporo)
Subject: Male, 74 years old
Diagnosis: Malignant lymphoma

Methodology & Outcome

This patient underwent surgery for an abdominal tumor in mid-1999. When the tumor could not be removed surgically, histological findings determined that the tumor was malignant lymphoma.

Chemotherapy was administered. There were strong side effects from the drug and the recommended dose could not be given at first. The tumor was found to persist in the CT scans and treatment was stopped. The patient was discharged in August.

A second opinion is when a patient seeks the advice of a second doctor when a treatment philosophy is unsatisfactory to the patient or there is no improvement in the disease. If a disease is serious, it is important to confirm the diagnosis, to confirm that the treatment method is appropriate, and to assess the risks of treatment by consulting a number of doctors.

Soon after his release, he consulted this clinic for treatment with AHCC and Chinese herbal medicine. The patient had suffered a loss of appetite from the anticancer drugs and he was experiencing profound weakness immediately after his initial discharge. He was very anemic, with low blood protein. The first recommendation was to use diet to recover his physical strength. AHCC and the Chinese herbal medicine Ginseng and Dang Gui Ten were prescribed. Although Etoposide (an anticancer drug) had been prescribed, since the tumor had persisted in the previous treatment, the patient refused it. He recovered his physical strength gradually and the tumor had nearly disappeared in a CT scan performed a year later. After two years, the tumor was clinically determined to have been eradicated.

Malignant lymphoma is roughly divided into Hodgkin's lymphoma and non-Hodgkin's lymphoma. In Japan, the frequency of occurrence of non-Hodgkin's lymphoma is high. Non-Hodgkin's lymphoma is further divided into B cell lymphoma and T cell lymphoma. In many cases, lymphoma of the neck, armpit, and groin can be self-diagnosed by the patient. If the disease develops and the focus of the disease spreads, treatment is difficult and the prognosis is considered to be bad. However, it can be cured by chemotherapy and radiation.

He has now recovered his physical strength through a regimen of balanced diet and exercise. He is enjoying tennis, traveling in the summer, and is enjoying an energetic lifestyle beyond expectation for a seventy-four-year old man.

AHCC IMPROVES QOL

QOL (Quality of Life) is a concept that emphasizes the patient's subjective experience of life as the most important aspect of treatment and not just the visible treatment results, such as tumor size. This encompasses maintaining and improving a patient's ease and comfort of mind and body as much as possible. In the past, QOL was often ignored in the treatment of cancer. In many cases, the reduction in QOL can mean decreased immune strength and low vitality. Aiming at improving the QOL has become the actual foundation of cancer treatment in more than seven hundred medical facilities in Japan.

It has already been noted that AHCC reduces side effects of anticancer drugs and radiation. This also improves a patient's QOL, regardless of whether or not the patient is undergoing chemotherapy or radiation. As the cancer progresses, patients often experience loss of appetite, pain, and discomfort in various parts of the body, plus mental distress and fatigue. There are many cases of cancer patients who have actually seen an improvement in their appetite, less pain, and regained their vitality soon after starting to take AHCC (see Figures 4.2 [page 85] and 4.7).

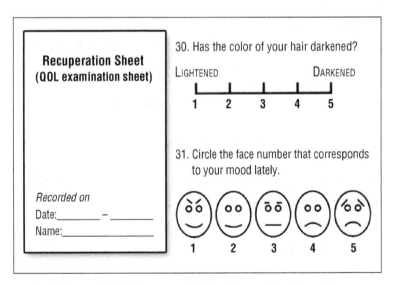

Figure 4.7 Quality of Life Patient Survey Questionnaire
for patients using AHCC

It may be considered an unorthodox opinion, but among doctors who are enthusiastic about alternative treatment, some say that it's good if a person can lead a vigorous and extended life without pain even if he is suffering from cancer. Cancer is a disease that becomes more curable when someone has a positive attitude and maintains a healthy lifestyle. Thus it can be said that raising the QOL is the primary role of cancer treatment, and AHCC is the most reliable health food for this purpose.

Cases in which AHCC had an evident effect in improving the QOL of terminal cancer patients are introduced below.

Researcher: Dr. Kenshiro Sugimoto, Sugimoto Clinic (Osaka)
Subject: Female, 45 years old
Diagnosis: Ovarian cancer

Methodology & Outcome

Ovarian cancer was diagnosed in a forty-five-year-old woman at Osaka R Hospital in December 1999, and the patient subsequently underwent a total hysterectomy. However, lymph node infiltrations in the pelvic basin and peritoneum, in which cancer cells from the ovary entered neighboring lymph nodes, were not removed and she was prescribed six courses of chemotherapy. By 2000, there was no change in the swelling of the inguinal (groin) lymph nodes. There was actually an increase in the size of the nodes, which prompted her to request a consultation at this clinic in May 2001. At the time of the consultation, she was being given a narcotic drug (MS Contin 60mg/day) for the pain.

The details of AHCC were explained to her at the time of the first medical examination and a regimen of twelve capsules of AHCC (around 6g) per day was started. At first she had swelling in the lower limbs, due to metastasis in the inguinal lymph nodes, followed by ascites (abdominal fluid accumulation). She was in constant pain, unable to sleep at night, and she had difficulty swallowing food. However, the family observed that after taking AHCC she became cheerful, could sleep soundly at night, and was able to eat soft food. The patient's daughter and son-in-law, who were taking care of her, were relieved.

Edema of the lower extremities tended to decrease after starting AHCC. Gradually, the lymphatic edema in the lower limbs went down considerably. The patient recovered from an almost bedridden state and was extremely happy that she could eat and even walk. She had a bigger smile every time she came in for a consultation and always went home laughing.

On August 8, 2001, she was sleeping at home, and around dawn woke her sleeping daughter, complaining about being bothered by the noise of the trains. She then went back to sleep. When her daughter woke up two hours later, her mother seemed to have stopped breathing. On the previous day, although she had complained of a backache, pain in the lower left leg, and vomiting, she had not increased the dose of the narcotic drug and had enjoyed the company of her family until eight hours before her death.

In this case, although the duration of taking AHCC was short, the onset of malignant peritonitis (peritonitis carcinomatosa) was delayed, there was reduction in the lymphatic edema in the lower limbs, the dosage of analgesic drugs (painkillers) was reduced, apprehensions about the struggle against the disease had eased, and the patient literally passed away in her sleep.

It has become very difficult to continue treatment in hospitals in the case of terminal cancer. *Home care* means receiving nursing care at home after being discharged from the hospital. This includes *home treatment* as well. How to continue treatment at home is a big problem in the case of cancer. In fact, home care is ideal; there is an overwhelming number of cases of death after transfer to the hospital.

Researcher: Dr. Kenshiro Sugimoto, Sugimoto Clinic (Osaka)
Subject: Female, 62 years old
Diagnosis: Breast cancer

Methodology & Outcome

A sixty-two-year-old female underwent surgery for cancer on the left breast in 1993. Subsequently, she took 600mg of the anti-cancer drug UFT. In 2000, she was diagnosed with rib metastasis from the breast cancer and underwent radiation therapy. She was also taking 10mg of MS Contin because of severe pain in the metastatic costal (rib) region.

She consulted the physicians of this hospital on the June 18, 1998, and was diagnosed with radiation esophagitis. In response, oral medication was administered. A persistent cough continued until September and pleural effusion, a buildup of fluid in the sac surrounding the left lung, was noticed in the x-ray examination, so 125ml of fluid was drained by puncture. In October, she had strongly hoped to attend her class reunion in South Korea, but had to abandon her travel plans since the breast cancer had affected the pleural membranes.

Her respiratory ailments were alleviated when a regimen of twelve capsules of AHCC (around 3g) was started, along with pleural drainage. She decided to reinstate her plans to travel to South Korea, and later safely returned home with wonderful memories and deepened connections to old friends. Although there was no increase in the pleural effusion for a while after returning home, she was hospitalized at the end of the year until the following February, due to a cold and difficulty breathing. While a small amount of pleural effusion was noticed after she was discharged from the hospital, she had no symptoms and continued to live well. Five-mm skin metastases were found in three places on the left side of the chest in August and were removed under local anesthesia.

Thereafter, although puncture draining was required around once a month, there was no pain specific to cancer and she regularly went to the hospital from her own house on foot. In November, regular visits to the hospital became very difficult, due to cold weather, and she was hospitalized again. There was no increase in the pleural effusion, even after hospitalization, and she would walk around the hospital and continued to live without any pain. In January 2002 she had a cardiac arrest immediately after returning to her bed from her usual walk. Although she was resuscitated right away, she could not talk much. Meanwhile, her husband was called and he came to the hospital. When he talked to her, she could not open her eyes, but she asked him to "Convey my regards and gratitude to all those who have cared for me," and passed away.

In this case, AHCC appeared to suppress the pleural effusion and extend her life for over two years after breast cancer bone metastasis was diagnosed. A remarkable improvement in QOL, including relieving cancer pain, was also observed. On visiting her husband a few days after he returned, we asked him, "Were your wife's last days comfortable?" The husband looked at the ground for a while and then with a relieved expression said, "Yes. She breathed her last as she had lived—very calm and quietly."

Accumulation of peritoneal fluid means that cancer or blood constituents have spread into the abdomen, leading to a massive breakdown of cells. This usually occurs at the end stage of cancer. Since the patient is in pain, fluid is removed by puncturing with a needle (called an abdominal tap), but it is only a temporary measure.

AHCC FOR NAUSEA, VOMITING, AND PAIN

The number-one side effect that cancer patients complain about during chemotherapy is vomiting. Second is hair loss, and third is nausea. Many times, chemotherapy, which holds the promise of being effective, is discontinued due to the severity of these side effects.

Dr. G. H. Ahn of South Korea's Ok-Cherm Hospital prescribed AHCC to twelve patients medically judged to have stage III–IV cancer for a period of eight months and then observed the changes in vomiting, nausea, and pain. He collected and analyzed data based on a unique checklist and confirmed that there was remarkable improvement in vomiting, nausea, and pain of the patients studied (see Figure 4.8).

Vomiting, pain, and nausea do not just cause discomfort and agony. They are acute stresses on the mind and body, which inhibit immune strength and vitality. Reducing these side

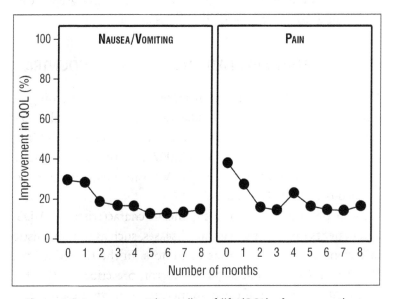

Figure 4.8 Improvement in quality of life (QOL) of cancer patients from administration of AHCC

effects through AHCC does more than merely alleviate suffering; it can also signify a greater possibility of a successful treatment outcome.

AHCC FOR RECOVERY OF APPETITE AND PREVENTION OF APPETITE LOSS

Appetite decrease due to chemotherapy causes the body to break down in many cases. Patients weaken and their condition deteriorates. AHCC is being used by many medical institutions, and many cancer patients have reported a reduction in the loss of appetite caused by the anticancer drugs. This is an extremely important effect of AHCC. With the increase in appetite, cancer patients regain lost weight and their general body condition and immune strength also increase.

AHCC seems to almost completely reduce the side effects of anticancer drugs. Radiation therapy also causes side effects similar to those of anticancer drugs and it is believed that AHCC can also be used to reduce these side effects as well.

REPORTS ABOUT AIDS PATIENTS IN FOREIGN COUNTRIES

The number of AIDS patients increases every year. According to estimates from the UNAIDS 2008 Report on the global AIDS epidemic, around 30.8 million adults and 2 million children were living with HIV at the end of 2007. According to the latest available statistics, the number of HIV-positive patients in Japan reached over 10,000 in 2007.

Decrease in immunity is a significant characteristic of AIDS, and patients can contract various diseases, such as opportunistic infections, and become prone to tumors. In the United States, Dr. Daniel Rubin, a naturopathic doctor, prescribed AHCC for AIDS patients and confirmed an increase in B-lymphocytes and CD8+ (immunity-related lymphocytes) (43,500–69,100). The possibility of preventing the drop in immunity increases with the use of AHCC.

Research is also under way at the Royal Hospital of Thailand using AHCC in nearly thirty AIDS patients. Plans call for examining the action of AHCC against AIDS by means of QOL improvement action and various immunological tests.

CURRENT INCIDENCE OF HEPATITIS IN JAPAN

In Japan, it is estimated that there are between 1 million and 2 million people with chronic hepatitis. Several types of hepatitis virus—A, B, C, and D—have been confirmed. Among the hepatitis patients, 20 percent are cases of hepatitis B virus and 70 percent are cases of hepatitis A virus. Approximately 90 percent of the chronic hepatitis patients develop the disease due to the hepatitis virus.

Some of the cases of B or C type of hepatitis virus advance to liver cirrhosis and from cirrhosis they degenerate into hepatocellular carcinoma (HCC). There are many cases in which the virus is not eliminated even with interferon treatment. Chronic viral hepatitis exemplifies a disease that is difficult to treat with modern medicine.

In diagnostic testing, first the blood is collected and antibodies or antigens are searched for. In the B-type virus, the HBs antigen becomes active; in the C type, the HCV antigen becomes active. Chronic liver dysfunction and hepatitis further lead to liver cell fibrosis, which changes to cirrhosis.

At this time the blood tests show high values of the liver enzymes GOT and GPT, indicating necrosis of the liver. The value of albumin (Alb) in the blood decreases as the protein synthesis ability is lowered due to functional liver failure. There is a correlation between the development of chronic hepatitis and a decrease in the number of platelets, which are important in the blood-clotting mechanism.

One of the complications of liver cirrhosis is liver cancer (HCC). The tumor markers alpha-fetoprotein (AFP) and PIV-KA-II are commonly used to diagnose this cancer. Nowadays hepatitis can be evaluated to some extent by thorough study of these test values.

AHCC FOR HEPATITIS PATIENTS

The action of AHCC on the liver was examined by covariance tests of hepatitis patients. It has been confirmed in some cases that when AHCC is taken by hepatitis and liver cancer patients, the decrease in the number of platelets is controlled, the viral load is decreased or eliminated, and deterioration of liver function is arrested. Even though there are a large number of reports of clinical observations on the effects of AHCC on patients with chronic liver diseases, the report by Dr. M. Iwamoto of Nobuyama Medical Corporation is introduced below as a representative example.

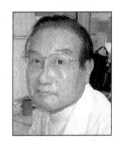

Researcher: Dr. M. Iwamoto, Nobuyama Medical Corporation (Sapporo)
Subject: Male, 32 years old
Diagnosis: Chronic hepatitis B

Methodology & Outcome

When AHCC (3g/day) was taken by a thirty-two-year-old male with chronic hepatitis B, the HBe antigen value (the indicator that shows the existing amount of the hepatitis B virus) decreased, and the HBe antibody value (the antibody that acts to eliminate the hepatitis B virus) increased. In addition, the elimination of the hepatitis B virus was confirmed (see Figure 4.9).

At the time this patient started taking AHCC, the value of AFP was 1,380ng/ml, which is well over the normal value of 20ng/ml.

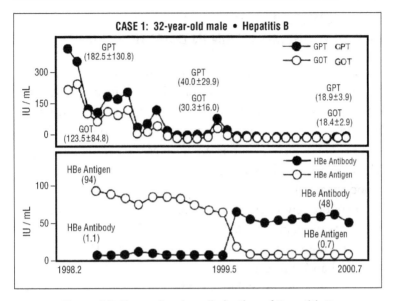

Figure 4.9 Charts showing elimination of Hepatitis B

After two months, the value had decreased to 800 and it continued to decrease until it reached a single digit, and this level was sustained. Although the platelet count decreased even after the patient started taking AHCC, it did not continue to decrease. Because of this and because the tumor marker value was kept in the normal range, it appears to be possible to prevent deterioration of the liver with AHCC in hepatitis patients.

The GOT and GPT values fluctuate dramatically in active hepatitis, particularly in the initial stages. There are people who believe that the GOT and GPT values increased because of AHCC. However, this is not the case. Normally, the GOT and GPT values become stable after several years. At that time, appropriate tests and diagnosis are necessary to judge whether the chronic hepatitis has changed to liver cirrhosis or is headed toward recovery.

AHCC LOWERS BLOOD SUGAR
AND GLYCOHEMOGLOBIN IN DIABETIC PATIENTS

Blood sugar levels of diabetic patients undergo many changes, depending on changing conditions. It is difficult to judge the effect of a treatment only by measuring blood sugar. Glyco-hemoglobin (HbA1c), which is formed by the bonding of sugar and hemoglobin, does not break down as rapidly as blood sugar. These numeric values reflect a one- to two-month average of blood sugar values.

Therefore, glycohemoglobin test values are a more depend-able measure than the standard glucose tolerance test. Generally, there is a high risk of disease complication if the HbA1c value is greater than 7.4 percent.

Dr. M. Iwamoto of Nobuyama Medical Corporation measured the blood sugar and glycohemoglobin values of thirteen diabetic patients who took AHCC for more than six months. As seen in Figure 4.10, the values of blood sugar and glycohemoglobin both

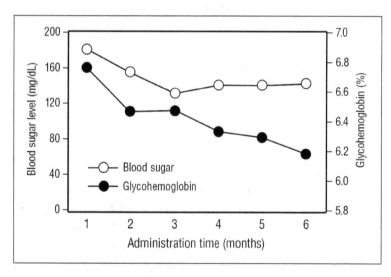

Figure 4.10 Change in the blood sugar and glycohemoglobin
values of patients taking AHCC

decreased and there was a remarkable decrease in the HbA1c values. Because HbA1c gets deposited on internal organs, it is the causative agent of complications such as kidney failure and cataracts. Prevention and reduction of these complications can be expected from taking AHCC.

USE OF AHCC FOR DIABETIC PATIENTS

According to the reports of Dr. Iwamoto, when AHCC is given to a patient whose blood sugar level before taking AHCC was 250mg/dl (normal value is 70–110) and the HbA1c value was 9.1 percent, the blood sugar level returned to a normal value and glycohemoglobin dropped to 6.8 percent after six months.

In a patient whose glycohemoglobin value had dropped to 6 percent within one month of starting AHCC, the blood sugar level also decreased to a normal value after two months. After that, normal values of glycohemoglobin were maintained, and there was also improvement in the paralysis of the left leg caused by diabetic neuropathy.

MORE AHCC CASE HISTORIES

We have reported numerous examples of improvement in cancer patients who are using AHCC. Among these are patients who survived terminal-stage cancer. However, since modern medicines and alternative medicines were used together in most cases, it is difficult to assess the effect of AHCC itself. Here are several cases in which the role of AHCC was clearly evident.

This book focuses on the "science of AHCC." However, many phenomena occur during actual clinical trials that cannot be scientifically verified. Though such phenomena may be only impressions or subjective experiences, they can be good news for some patients.

These are examples related to the action of AHCC that were

actually reported by the AHCC Study Group, an informal group that collects impressions and experiences with AHCC from patients, health care professionals, and third person observers.

A Doctor Who Struggled with His Own Stomach Cancer

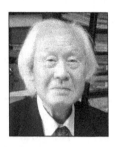

Dr. Masa Toki (eighty-nine years old), director of Toki Internal Medicine (Gumma Prefecture, Haruna City), practiced for many years with his son, also a physician, in that part of Japan. Even today, once or twice a week, he takes part in clinic activities, such as physical examinations, and works as a doctor on a panel of medical school physicians.

About ten years ago, he noticed something wrong. He found a polyp in his stomach by endoscopy and had it removed year after year. Since these polyps can be cancerous, he worked on preventing them by using immunostimulants and various health foods.

Stomach cancer was detected and was excised using a laser at the University Hospital. However, a recurrence was confirmed by endoscopy a year later and it was found that the cancer had penetrated to the muscular layer, as shown in Figure 4.11 (image at left). Surgery was not possible because of his age and physical condition. He began to take 3g/day of AHCC, along with an anticancer drug (UFT) and several types of health foods, which he had been taking for many years.

After one month it was found that the stomach cancer had shrunk considerably, as seen in Figure 4.11 (image at right). Moreover, the typical side effects of the anticancer drug were not apparent in the blood tests. Dr. Toki has said that this can be explained from the viewpoint of recent psychoneuroimmunology (psycho-oncology—see sidebar, page 115) research. For the past thirty-five years, he had engaged in voluntary service as a devout

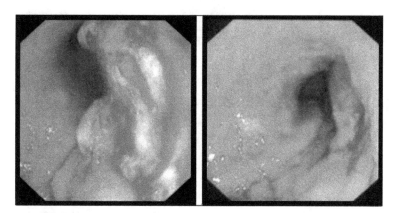

Figure 4.11 After one month of treatment with AHCC, it was found that the stomach cancer had shrunk considerably (right)

Christian in Japan as well as in other countries. Even after he learned that he had cancer, he had a firm belief that he was ready to go when summoned by God, and had practically no fear of death. Many believe that such a positive and worry-free state of mind can have a positive effect on immunity.

In 1950, research on psychological adaptation to cancer was carried out by a group of psychiatrists at Massachusetts General Hospital. They reported that change in the progression of cancer is correlated with a particular communication pattern. It was found that when patients with advanced cancer had limited communication skills, there was a strong tendency toward guilt feelings as a psychological reaction. This was the first thesis advanced about psychological reactions to cancer. Even though effective treatments for cancer were developed later, patients who overcame the side effects of this treatment still developed psychological problems. So a new field of study, called psycho-oncology, was developed within oncology. This branch studies the effect of emotions on the immune system and the endocrine system, and the relationship between the emotions and cancer risk.

His involvement with cancer may still continue and Dr. Toki, who is leading a positive and cheerful life as a doctor and a Christian, has expressed a wish to pass on his experience.

A Survivor of Terminal-Stage Pancreatic Cancer

A sixty-two-year-old man, a resident of Osaka, who managed a packing material company, complained of a backache in June 1995 and underwent tests in a nearby hospital. He was shifted to Government Hospital for a thorough checkup and was diagnosed with terminal-stage pancreatic cancer of the papilla (a small muscle located where the common bile duct empties into the duodenum) with kidney infiltration. The tests were carried out as he endured considerable back pain, and peritoneal fluid also accumulated after a few weeks. It was confirmed that he had reached a stage where nothing could be done. It was a remarkably urgent case, but neither surgery nor chemotherapy was possible.

One month later, his family obtained AHCC and through repeated efforts, they were gradually able to get him to swallow small amounts. After a few days, there was a complete change in his condition and he could take meals normally. Although he suffered a great deal of pain, after a few days of taking AHCC, he realized that his condition had improved and he could think about the disease in a calmer state of mind.

He researched many alternative treatments and decided to fight the cancer with the combined treatment of AHCC and other health foods or supplements and alternative treatments. He said that he would continue to take AHCC no matter what, while visualizing that his cancer was becoming smaller with the combined use of his intention and psychotherapy.

At that time, his doctor confirmed that there was no doubt that the progression of the cancer had stopped and was in remission. The patient underwent regular checkups in the hospital in June 1995, July 1995, May 1996, and March 1997 and the cancer was found to have diminished and finally completely disappeared.

By 2002, the patient had regained complete health and reported that family support, immunity-boosting health foods, intention, and the use of imagery were all important for maintaining health.

Figure 4.12 shows the photographic images immediately after the diagnosis in 1995 and the image after three years of taking AHCC.

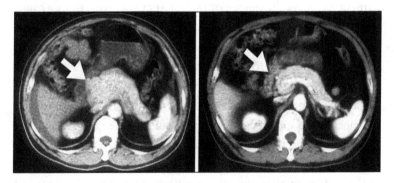

Figure 4.12 Photographic image immediately after the diagnosis in 1995 (left) and the image after three years of taking AHCC (right)

Experiences of a Cancer Patient

Toshiyuki Watanabe of Kokurakita Prefecture, sixty years old, underwent endoscopy in April 1999 in which four tumors were found. He was diagnosed with urinary bladder cancer (histological tissue sample tests were not carried out at that time). At that time he started taking 6g/day of AHCC and when he again underwent a thorough checkup after three weeks he found that the tumor had disappeared completely.

There has been no relapse to this date. Mr. Watanabe has talked to many patients about his own experiences with health foods. Examples of two patients who consulted Mr. Watanabe are given below.

1. A seventy-six-year-old man with esophageal cancer was hospitalized in a government hospital in October 2001. He didn't want to undergo the operation and therefore consulted Mr. Watanabe. On Mr. Watanabe's recommendation, he consulted the outpatient clinic of Dr. S. of Ogura Itozu Hospital. In the opinion of Dr. S., there was a tumor of approximately 3cm in the central thoracic esophagus. Among digestive tract cancers, esophageal cancer has high degree of lymph node metastasis. As the degree of malignancy was remarkably high, Dr. S. recommended surgery and radiation therapy. However, since the patient was not keen on the operation, he started taking AHCC (9g/day) and other health supplement drinks under the guidance of Dr. S. and Mr. Watanabe. On the third day after starting AHCC, an unpleasant feeling he experienced when he ate disappeared. He also started the radiation therapy, according to the instructions of Dr. S. After two months, the tumor disappeared and there were no side effects from the radiation therapy. He was discharged from the hospital in good health. He continues to be in good health and takes 2g/day of AHCC.

2. A seventy-eight-year-old man, living in Kitakyushu, was diagnosed with jaundice in March 1998. He was hospitalized and various tests were carried out. Although bile duct cancer was diagnosed at that time, surgery was not possible, since he had heart disease and kidney disease. After being hospitalized on and off, he consulted the Outpatient Clinic of Dr. S. of Ogura Itozu Hospital and underwent an abdominal CT and an echo test. A tumor of approximately 2cm diameter was found in the common bile duct below the gallbladder. The tumor marker (PIVKA II) had also increased to 4,194 (normal: less than 40). Treatment for this condition is difficult.

Since he wanted to try all possible treatments, he took AHCC with other health foods, as advised by Mr. Watanabe. His QOL improved and in few months there was improvement in the test values (as shown in Table 4.5). There was improvement of the jaundice and the quantity of AHCC was reduced to 3g/day.

TABLE 4.5 CASE OF MR. S. N., MALE, 78 YEARS OLD; DIAGNOSIS: COMMON BILE DUCT CANCER					
	NORMAL VALUES	2001 JUN 22	SEP 21	OCT 17	NOV 14	2002 JAN 25
Total bilirubin	0.2–1.1	3.4	4.8	1.6	1.0	0.3
GOT	10–40	179	165	54	37	26
GPT	5–45	143	85	22	22	16
γ-GPT	Below 75	648	483	156	103	26
PIVKA II	Less than 40	4194	8392	–	–	25

By January 2002 there was no change in the chronic heart disease or kidney disease, the tumor marker level (PIVKA II) normalized to 2.5, and there was slight anemia. Eight months after the start of the treatment, he was surprisingly healthy and still pursues his hobby of painting.

Mr. Watanabe drew from his own experience to help take care of the mental and physical needs of these patients without interfering with the doctor's treatment plan.

RECOMMENDATIONS FROM SPECIALISTS IN CHINESE MEDICINE

Some experts who prescribe AHCC use many experimental methodologies. Ideas related to cancer treatment with AHCC, as seen from the viewpoint of specialists, are introduced below.

Profile

Dr. Toru Morooka
Graduate of Iwate Medical University
Director, Morooka Internal Medicine Clinic
  (Sapporo, Japan)

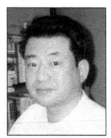

Dr. Morooka is a medical doctor who has
carried out extensive clinical research as a doctor of Chinese
medicine. Currently he is the director of the Morooka Internal
Medicine Clinic in Sapporo, Japan. He is a member of the Japanese Oriental Medicine Association and the Japanese Internal
Medicine Association.

Dr. Morooka studied Chinese medicine theory according to
the ancient classical Chinese medical literature and he treats
patients with a wide range of diseases at the Chinese Medicine
Prescription Center. He has been getting good results for years
with the combined use of AHCC and Chinese medicine on cancer
patients.

An important factor in Chinese medicine as it is practiced in
Japan is regulation of so-called "stomach energy." Controlling
the intake and discharge of this energy and circulating it in the
whole body without stagnation is considered to be the key to
good treatment results. This concept of preserving stomach energy, circulating it, and returning it to the center at just the right
time has been presented at AHCC Seminars held every year and
is in accord with many Western medicine concepts.

AHCC is used as a Chinese medicine when there is very little stomach energy and it cannot be regulated properly. In other
words, there is an imbalance because the stomach energy is completely depleted. AHCC works to restore the exhausted stomach
energy. AHCC is probably unsuitable for controlling problems
caused by excess stomach energy. However, AHCC alone does not
seem to be sufficient when there is a problem with the flow of
stomach energy. In these cases, combining AHCC with Chinese

> The concept of stomach energy in Chinese medicine is as follows: First, the food we eat is digested and converted into vital energy. This stomach energy is distributed throughout the body. It is also necessary for this energy not to be generated in excess. This concept is similar to the Western concept of immunity.

medicines should be considered. Several cases in which AHCC was used alone for an extended period, and appeared to be effective, are briefly described here as well.

1. **A case in which only AHCC was used.** An eighty-seven-year-old woman whose main complaint was a stomachache, was diagnosed with stomach cancer. Immunotherapy was decided on after discussion with family members. She was given 3g of AHCC per day and told that it was a stomach medicine. Since the stomachache disappeared instantly, she thought that the prescribed stomach medicine was very effective. In the endoscopy done three years after the start of the treatment, the tumor had disappeared. In this case, AHCC was thought to be effective for stomachache or tumor formation caused by insufficient stomach energy.

2. **A case in which AHCC and Cinnamon and Astragalus Combination were used together.** A fifty-seven-year-old female developed alveolar cell carcinoma from multiple metastases in the lungs after surgery for ovarian cancer. She came for a consultation with the intention of undergoing immunotherapy. She was treated with 3g of AHCC along with the traditional Chinese formula called Cinnamon and Poria Combination, but the effect was weak during the first year and the tumor in the lung gradually continued to grow. The tumor shrank when the Chinese medicine was changed to Cinnamon and Astragalus Combination. After one year, the tumor had disappeared completely, according to a chest x-ray. She was very happy and

was told to get a CT scan once a year. In this patient, stomach energy drained from the lung to the intestines with an adverse effect on the intestine. This was interpreted wrongly as a lung excess condition and the patient was given Cinnamon and Poria Combination. Since the herbal medicine was changed in time, it was effective for the patient.

Dr. Morooka treated his patients by individualizing the treatment for each person's unique type and selecting a Chinese herbal formula specifically for the patient's condition. Before treatment, he confirmed what other treatment the patient was undergoing and what treatment the patient should have, since certain health foods can be unsuitable for the body in some cases.

Chinese medicine is prescribed based on the individual signs and symptoms of the patient. Chinese medicine differs from Western medicine in this regard, since Western medicine is prescribed for cancer and not the individual's unique body type. Neither Cinnamon and Poria Combination nor Cinnamon and Astragalus Combination are specifically used for cancer, but the choice of these formulas was based on considerations of the patient's body type and set of symptoms. In this way Chinese medicine strives to choose the medication that is best suited for

In the latter half of the seventeenth century, the belief that the foundation of medical science and Confucianism were the same deepened. Authorities on the medical classics began to question this belief, reexamining their sense that these two ways of viewing life were somehow identical; this caused a revolution in thought. A new system was developed in Japan by collecting experimental case histories and using ancient Chinese systems (especially the *Shang Han Lun*). This school of thought is called the *Kohoha*, or "Ancient Methods School." It was divided further into two schools of thought in the middle of the Edo period (1603–1868).

the person's constitution, based on the evaluation of the Chinese medicine specialist.

A PHARMACIST WHO INTRODUCED AN ALTERNATIVE TREATMENT

Profile

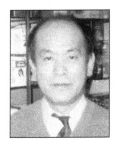

Pharmacist Sumitaka Ooura

Graduate of the Kyoto Pharmaceutical
   University

Managing Director of the Human Medicine
   Company (Ltd.) and Human Medicine
   Pharmacy (Osaka)

Managing Director of the Human Medicine Research Laboratory

Member of the Structural Medical Association of Japan and Integrative Medical Association of Japan

The Human Medicine Company (Ltd.) and the Human Medicine Pharmacy in Osaka are among the few pharmacies in Japan that specialize in complementary and alternative medicines. Mr. Ooura, who is a pharmacist, has counseled many people on a day-to-day basis. Historically, people have taken health advice from the town pharmacist as if he were their personal counselor. In Japan as well, the role of pharmacists has become more important in recent years. A prominent feature of the Human Medicine Company is the vast number of "rules of thumb" related to food and the human body acquired over the past sixty years. Mr. Ooura has been recommending AHCC as an immunostimulant health food to cancer patients from the time he was introduced to it.

Naturally, as patients visited the hospital and pharmacy, Mr. Ooura gave advice on health, especially advice concerning health foods and eating habits, so that patients could get the maximum benefit from treatment prescribed by their doctors. He says, "I always explain the theory of immunity of Professor Toru Abo of

Tohoku University to the people who come to me for counseling on cancer. Many people who have cancer are excessively hard-working people, people who suppress their emotions, or heavy drinkers. In women, they are often married women who have a troubled married life or other types of worries."

Professor Abo's hypothesis is that chronic stress strains the sympathetic nervous system. If the stress on the sympathetic nervous system is sustained, various symptoms, such as increased pulse rate, elevated blood pressure, high blood sugar levels, insomnia, shoulder stiffness and chronic fatigue manifest, but even more troubling are the obstructions in blood flow and increased numbers of granulocytes, which suppress the immune system.

The group of cells that defend our bodies from invasion by microorganisms or foreign bodies are the white blood cells, or lymphocytes. For these cells to work efficiently, the autonomic nervous system must be properly regulated. Granulocytes are under the control of the sympathetic nervous system, while lymphocytes are under the control of the parasympathetic nervous system. Professor Abo describes the control of white blood cells by autonomic nerves in this theory and it is regarded as a persuasive theory of the development of cancer.

Moreover, if excessive strain on sympathetic nerves continues, it damages tissues and internal organs, due to obstructions in the peripheral blood flow caused by dead cells and an increase in granulocytes. These obstructions exert a strong effect on epithelial cells of the skin and intestines. Since the epithelial cells of the skin and intestines are dynamic places with rapid cell turnover, the attack of granulocytes exerts a strong effect on them. If this continues over a long period, large quantities of active oxygen are generated as a result of the increased number of granulocytes. Cells are injured due to the strong oxidative action of this large volume of active oxygen. This could be the reason for the development of cancer, especially if these conditions induce the expression of a genetic defect.

The sympathetic and parasympathetic nerves have opposite influences in the body. If the sympathetic nervous system is dominant, natural killer (NK) T cells that attack cancer cells, which are under the control of parasympathetic nervous system, cannot function properly.

According to this model of cancer development, cancer immunotherapy should involve strengthening the activity of the parasympathetic nervous system to a considerable degree and dealing with stress more effectively. When the parasympathetic nervous system predominates, appetite is regained, bowel movements are improved, sleep patterns improve, and a relaxed state of mind results.

Although there are many medications called immunostimulants, an ideal treatment plan would stimulate parasympathetic predominance with products that best match the patient's needs. Among all these immunostimulants, I have observed that AHCC induces this type of response very effectively. Symptoms of parasympathetic nerve insufficiency, such as loss of appetite, insomnia, and fatigue, are eliminated in a short period among the cancer patients who respond well to AHCC. They regain their appetite, their sleep is restorative, and they ease into a relaxed state of mind—all signs of parasympathetic dominance.

One key role of health care workers is to advise patients so that these results can be achieved. Overall immunity is increased as a result of the activation of lymphocytes. A state of parasympathetic nerve dominance must be sustained in patients to obtain these results.

It is also important to advise the patient that a diet that is high in fiber, with a central focus on vegetables, is necessary to help suppress the effects of active oxygen. And, again, medical professionals must focus on the deleterious effects of stressful aspects of a person's life, such as overwork, excessive drinking, or excessive worry.

The Oriental medicine approach involves examining any reasons why cancer should exist. Cancer cells consume ten times more energy than normal cells, and they go on consuming this energy as long as they exist. From this standpoint, it is necessary to create a healthy lifestyle by discussing with the patient how to limit this excess energy. According to this theory, one of the factors that creates and supports cancer will disappear if this excessive energy can be controlled.

REPUTATION OF AHCC IN OTHER COUNTRIES

AHCC has attracted a lot of attention internationally. The expectations of AHCC are increasing, especially as the body of peer-reviewed literature on its use and efficacy grows. Here are comments from a couple of experts.

Profile

Dr. Francisco Contreras
Director of Oasis Hospital (Tijuana, Mexico)
Consults for other hospitals in treatment focused on
    complementary and alternative medicine

While these mushrooms have been cited in ancient Japanese texts as a source of increased immunity, there are no reports on whether products extracted from these mushrooms are effective in treating cancer patients, whose immunity is lowered because of chemotherapy.

Dr. Francisco Contreras felt that a thorough evaluation of the immunostimulating action of AHCC extracted from mushrooms on cancer patients with low immunity caused by chemotherapy is necessary not only for cancer patients but for cancer experts as well. So he performed research in conjunction with Amino Up Chemical Company and Oasis Hospital (Oasis of Hope Hospital, Tijuana, Mexico).

old, half of a 500mg capsule of AHCC is given twice a day in the initial stages of viral infection. If the symptoms are considerably advanced, one capsule can be given twice a day. AHCC is also effective for severe symptoms if the intake quantity is increased. He has used Chinese medicines and pediatric acupuncture for treatment of acute infections, but these treatments are not necessary in most cases when AHCC is used.

In the case of infectious diseases in adults, he gives AHCC in larger quantities and has seen effects similar to those in children. He especially recommends AHCC to patients who are taking antibiotics to prevent the recurrence of the infection. His philosophy is to treat the patient with Chinese medicine and AHCC to avoid using antibiotics, if at all possible.

In the future he plans to implement AHCC in the treatment of hepatitis. He believes that the treatment will be extremely effective if AHCC and Chinese medicine are used together. Neither AHCC nor Chinese medicines are widely known among mainstream U.S. medical practitioners. Kenner hopes that Japa... scientists will blaze the trail for the use of AHCC for h... the results are good, it will lead to a treatmen... at regeneration of the liver and the imm... an attempt to kill the virus.

Dr. Contreras designed double-blind, placebo-controlled tests in a population of patients with immunity lowered as a result of chemotherapy. The patients were divided into two groups. One group was given a placebo and the other was given AHCC. The group that was given AHCC showed substantial resilience to the effects of the anticancer drugs, and there was a distinct diminution in the occurrence and severity of side effects from those drugs.

Dr. Contreras had never come across a product that yielded such good results in precise clinical trials. He was convinced that AHCC not only protected and activated immunity, but that it was also useful in strengthening the immune system as an adjuvant to treatment (a substance that activates antibody production and the immune response). It is also an effective measure as a primary therapy not only for cancer, but for any disease that compromises immunity.

AHCC plays an important role in reducing the side effects of chemotherapy like nausea, lethargy, and hair loss.

Profile

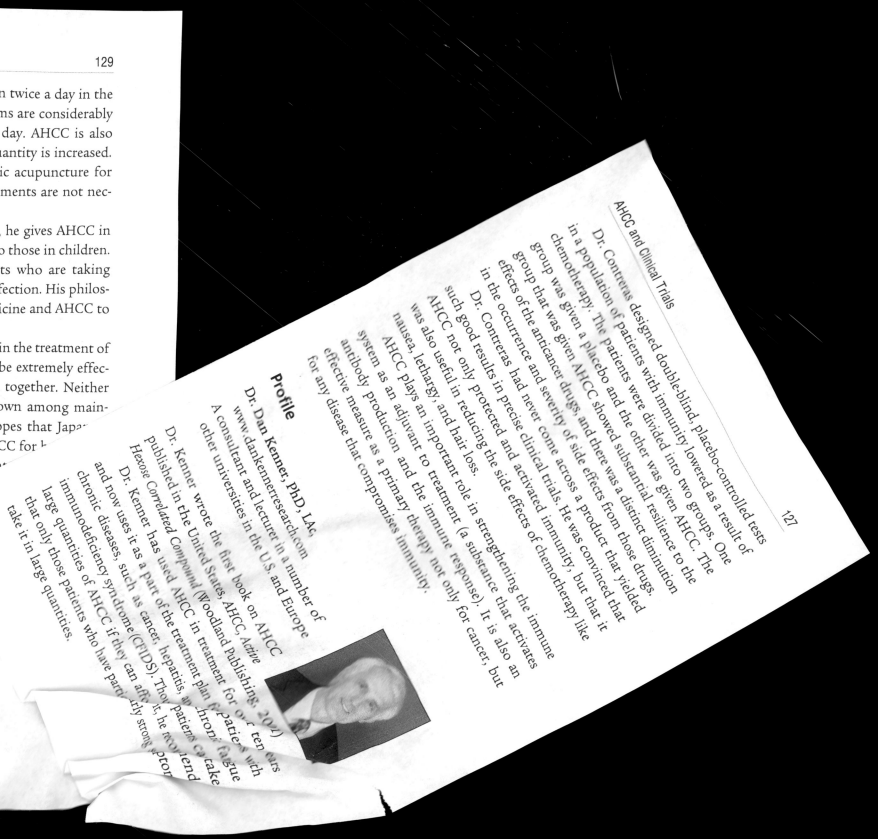

Dr. Dan Kenner, PhD, LAc
www.dankennerresearch.com
A consultant and lecturer in a number of other universities in the U.S. and Europe

Dr. Kenner wrote the first book on AHCC published in the United States, *AHCC, Active Hexose Correlated Compound* (Woodland Publishing, 2001)

Dr. Kenner has used AHCC as a part of the treatment plan for patients with chronic diseases, such as cancer, hepatitis, and now uses it as a part of the treatment... patients c... take immunodeficiency syndrome (CFIDS). Tho... he recommend large quantities of AHCC if they can affo... it, that only those patients who have particularly strong sympto... take it in large quantities.

He recommends 4.5–6.0 g/day for cancer patients for ten to twelve weeks; after that, he advises them to decrease the amount to 3g/day. For fatigue syndrome, he recommends 3g/day of AHCC for at least six weeks.

Dr. Kenner reports having seen a marked increase in the level of NK cell activity in a patient with advanced ovarian cancer, which convinced him of its value. Patients with chronic fatigue often make remarkable recoveries, even though often less than the recommended dose is necessary. Long-term treatment for hepatitis patients is necessary. Though rapid recovery can be seen in the immune system, it takes time to confirm changes in the liver condition. He feels that it is definitely worth their while to take AHCC as directed, because the results are consistent. Kenner says that the therapeutic properties of the healing mushrooms of Japan are well known in America, and there are some products that are much more expensive than AHCC but not nearly as effective. AHCC is the most effective and economical option.

When he was introduced to AHCC, he observed its remarkable effect on the cellular-mediated (Th1) immune system. He thought at first that positive effects of AHCC could not be expected in cases of acute infection and allergies because it acts only on the Th1-regulated immunity. He found this to be a very rigid concept. He used it for his own symptoms of allergic rhinitis (hay fever) in the period of late spring to the early summer and the effect of AHCC was very dramatic. Symptoms such as irritation of eyes, a feverish feeling and a runny nose stop...

...fever even than a pharmaceutical drug. Th...

...American product is a gelatin...

...was strained for three days...

...mild, he becam...

CHAPTER 5

Questions and Answers about AHCC

ROLE OF AHCC IN CANCER TREATMENT

All information on AHCC is in the form of Questions and Answers in this chapter. Although some of the information has already been covered in other parts of the book, the Q&A format should be useful as a concise summary of what we know about AHCC. All the answers are from summaries of reports or from excerpts of discussions of the AHCC Society.

What are alternative medical treatments?
Treatments that use folk medicines or folk remedies as opposed to medical treatments based on Western medicine are generally called alternative medical treatments (or just "alternative treatments"). Associations to investigate and evaluate scientific evidence of alternative medical treatments have been established in Japan. Alternative medical treatments are not necessarily incompatible with Western medicine. There has also been a rapid rise in the formation of medical treatment systems known as integrative, or complementary, medical treatment, in which the alternative medical treatments and Western medicine complement each other.

What kinds of methods are available for cancer immunotherapy?

There is a wide range of methods for treating cancer, including medical treatments, such as adoptive immunotherapy, in which the lymphocytes are activated and then administered to cancer patients along with mind-body therapies. Immunotherapy, using drugs (immune stimulants) and health foods, plus immunotherapies based on psychological and emotional support, are among the many methods of cancer treatment. Since AHCC is a health food, it can also be called an alternative treatment, which can be safely used by anyone. AHCC has been on the horizon since its immunological activation effects were scientifically and medically confirmed by the AHCC Research Association, established in 1994. Although it has not been approved (certified) as a pharmaceutical medicine, AHCC and other comparable alternative treatments have been attracting attention as supplemental adjuncts to modern medical treatment.

Is there a possibility that AHCC will be approved (certified) as a pharmaceutical medicine in the near future?

The AHCC Research Association has come to the conclusion that AHCC must remain classified as a health food to make the best use of its wide-ranging properties. If it were to be classified as a pharmaceutical, that would tend to limit its widespread use. It has been confirmed by research that the effects of AHCC are obtained from high-quality, reliable raw materials. The manufacturing equipment used to make AHCC also meets the manufacturing standards of pharmaceuticals. The reason for not seeking pharmaceutical certification for AHCC has nothing to do with the standards of its manufacture or quality control. AHCC can be used safely by people with a variety of conditions and ailments, and as a preventive, so it was decided that AHCC must be categorized as a health food.

RELATIONSHIP BETWEEN AHCC
AND MEDICAL TREATMENTS

Why is a statement of efficacy not provided on health foods like AHCC?

The obvious difference between health foods and drugs is that the effects of drugs can be stated legally. Even if a lot of medical data is put together to prove the effectiveness of a health food, it is illegal to label it with any statement regarding its efficacy.

Are there doctors who have not given their seal of approval to AHCC?

Many doctors do not use health foods like AHCC for immuno-therapy. The reasons for this may be that the effects of treatments not covered by health insurance have probably not been judged accurately and data on the medical rationale for using health foods is not readily available. Regrettably, some health food–related businesses have also been the source of animosity between the health food industry and the medical establishment. Under normal circumstances, it is best if AHCC is taken with the consent and under the supervision of a doctor. However, since it is believed that health foods do not hinder medical treatment or the effects of drugs if taken in appropriate amounts, the final decision about whether or not to take the health food rests solely with patients themselves.

What if I wish to refuse surgery and chemotherapy and take only AHCC?

Modern medical diagnosis and medical treatments are indis-pensable in cancer treatment. Patients should take it upon themselves to learn everything they can about their disease and decide on the course of treatment after proper consultation with a doctor.

AHCC RESEARCH IN MEDICAL INSTITUTIONS

What kinds of institutions are involved in AHCC research?

AHCC research is carried out not only in Japan but also in medical institutions and university medical research facilities in the United States, China, Korea, and Thailand. These medical institutes are reporting not only animal test results but also effects of AHCC with actual cancer patients.

To what extent has the AHCC data been made public?

AHCC data has basically been presented in scientific conferences and published research papers. Besides these, information about AHCC can be found in various books and lectures by experts (see Suggestions for Further Reading at the end of this book and www.ahccpublishedresearch.com).

Are university hospitals using AHCC?

AHCC is being used in ten universities from Hokkaido to Kyushu for clinical trials and also at numerous research institutions, including Yale University, Drexel University, University of California at Davis, and M.D. Anderson Cancer Center of the University of Texas in the United States; the Ok-Cherm Hospital in Korea; Southern China Agricultural University in China; and the National Cancer Institute in Thailand.

AHCC MANUFACTURING

What are the mushrooms that are used as the raw material for AHCC?

The thready mycelia, which are like the mushrooms' roots, are cultures. There are several types of mushrooms that are hybridized with shiitake (*Lentinus edodes*) to make the mushroom culture.

In what form are AHCC products available?

AHCC products are available as fine granules, soft granules in capsules, and as a liquid. Since all types are for oral intake, AHCC cannot be administered by injection. The form of the product can be selected according to one's preference. Since AHCC is manufactured only by the Amino Up Chemical Company, there are no concerns about the variations in the quality.

Since enzyme reactions are used in the AHCC manufacturing process, do the AHCC products contain any of those enzymes?

Although enzyme reactions are used in the manufacturing process of AHCC, the enzyme activity disappears in the later stages of the process and, as such, there are no enzymes in the AHCC product. The purpose of using enzyme reactions is to break down the hard cell walls of the hyphae (fungus threads) of the basidiomycetes, the raw material of AHCC, and to extract the active constituents from inside the basidiomycete cells. The enzymes have an indispensable function in the manufacturing of AHCC because they break down large molecules into smaller ones and, to a certain extent, the active constituent polysaccharides are low molecular weight molecules.

When I bought AHCC recently, why did I feel that the color and smell were different from previous AHCC products I'd purchased?

Since AHCC is made from cultures of mushrooms, it is difficult to keep manufacturing exactly the same product, as with chemicals. However, the AHCC manufacturing plant has acquired international standard accreditations, such as the HACCP and ISO9002, as explained in chapter 1. The equipment used in the Amino Up plants matches the equipment used for manufacturing pharmaceuticals. AHCC is manufactured with such thorough quality control that it can be said to be extremely consistent in quality.

CONSTITUENTS OF AHCC

What are the plant polysaccharides that form the main constituents of AHCC?

Several monosaccharides (such as glucose) are connected in a chain to form a polysaccharide. Although monosaccharides are easy-to-absorb energy sources, polysaccharides are generally more difficult to digest and difficult to absorb as energy. On the other hand, polysaccharides demonstrate salient effects, such as stimulating important vital processes in the body and improving immunity (see chapter 1).

Explain the AHCC constituents in detail.

AHCC contains various vitamins and minerals in small quantities, but the polysaccharides make up about 44 percent of the total constituents (see Table 1.2 for detailed constituent percentages). These polysaccharides include β-glucan and α-glucan. Both act to improve cell-mediated immunity. It is believed that the key to the immunological activity of AHCC lies in the acetylated α-glucan.

Is it true that health foods that contain low molecular weight, water-soluble constituents are the most effective?

Many health foods are touted as "highly water-soluble" and "low molecular weight." Although highly water-soluble and low molecular weight constituents are generally considered to be effective and easy to absorb, this reasoning does not always hold true. Most Western medicines are made of constituents that do not dissolve easily in water, but are properly absorbed in the body. Evidently, constituents that do not have a low molecular weight cannot be absorbed, but the high molecular weight β-glucan is believed to stimulate "gut immunity," even though it is difficult to absorb. Although there are many water-soluble, low molecular weight constituents in AHCC, very little is known about how they are absorbed and act inside the body. A detailed mechanism of action of AHCC is yet to be elucidated, but its reliability has been proved by the abundant data that has been collected about its actual use.

What is the major difference between AHCC and other mushroom products?

Let's list the differences between AHCC and other mushroom products:

- Only one company manufactures AHCC and, as such, there are no variations in its quality.

- In AHCC, the mushroom bacteria are cultured in tanks for long time periods and the unique constituent acetylated α-1,4 glucan is produced.

- There has been a lot of clinical research on AHCC and a lot of data about its efficacy has been generated.

Are there any changes in a person's physical condition that result when he or she starts to take AHCC?

It is reported that there is an improvement in quality of life (QOL) within a few days to a few weeks after starting AHCC. Improvements in appetite and sleep patterns, and a diminution in the side effects of anticancer drugs have all been confirmed to occur relatively soon. Pain relief and life extension have also been reported in cancer patients. Scientific data from hospital tests reveal that the immune indices in the blood increase within a few months of starting AHCC. There have been reports of eczema and itching, but their relation to the action of AHCC is not clear. Generally, such reactions do not lead to serious side effects and it is believed that these reactions disappear over time.

HOW TO TAKE AHCC

Are there any other health foods or medicines that are incompatible with taking AHCC?

AHCC is a health food and there are no problems even if it is taken along with conventional medicines, such as anticancer drugs, interferon, insulin, and the like. There are no reports of side effects. As long as it is taken in appropriate quantities, combining it with other health foods should not pose any problems. In any event, it is recommended that AHCC should be used after proper consultation with the prescribing physician if a patient is taking prescription drugs.

Are there any health foods that combine particularly well with AHCC?

Many patients taking AHCC—especially cancer patients—combine it with other health foods, supplements, and alternative treatments, even with Western medical treatment. Each person has to make the decision about choosing suitable health foods to combine with AHCC. Antioxidant vitamins (like vitamin C and vitamin E) or minerals that are indispensable to the body are readily available and compatible with AHCC. It would be irresponsible to say that cancer can be completely cured solely with AHCC. The possibility of recovery from cancer depends greatly on what type of cancer the patient has and the stage of the cancer, as well as the patient's age and disposition. However, it is probably a good idea to augment AHCC by combining it with other health foods and supplements with a variety of functions, rather than simply taking several kinds of mushroom-based health foods.

What are the proper dose and method of taking AHCC?

If the purpose is prevention or health maintenance, 1-3g of AHCC daily (or two to six 500mg capsules a day) is appropriate.

The intake quantity should be 3g per day to prevent recurrence of cancer, and 3-6g per day during cancer treatment. In both cases, it is recommended that the amount of AHCC be divided and taken three times a day. Since there is no problem with taking it along with anticancer drugs or radiation therapy, 3-6g per day of AHCC should be taken before starting chemotherapy. These dosage levels have been released by the AHCC Research Association on the basis of the experiences of doctors who have prescribed AHCC. Of course, taking AHCC at the recommended dosage does not guarantee a cure.

Is there any problem if a healthy person takes AHCC?

No problem at all. In fact, it is believed that the antioxidant properties of AHCC can prevent cancer and other chronic or lifestyle-related diseases. The dosage of 3-6g per day of AHCC is suitable for cancer patients, but 1-3g per day is sufficient for a healthy person for health maintenance.

How should we administer AHCC to children and elderly people?

In the case of children, the dosage can be reduced by up to half because of lower body weight. In elderly people, it is important to moderate the dose to match their physical condition, since they may have weak stomachs. In either case, AHCC can be mixed with yogurt or honey.

Are there individual variations in the effects of AHCC?

There may be individual differences in sensing the effects of AHCC, depending on one's age, the body's constitution, and whether one is sick. It can be said of all mushroom-based health foods that they do not necessarily increase the immunity of everyone who takes them. However, most people have confirmed an improvement in QOL; for example, there is often improvement in appetite within about a week of taking AHCC. It is necessary to measure the changes in the blood tests of immunity to ascertain these individual variations scientifically.

How long should a person take AHCC?

This question is often asked by people after surgery. AHCC should be taken for as long as possible to prevent any recurrence, especially if the patient has had cancer. For health maintenance, patients should judge according to their personal sense of well-being.

Has the safety of AHCC been confirmed?

Acute toxicity tests were conducted on animals to verify the safety of AHCC. The tests were carried out according to GLP (Good Laboratory Practice; that is, safety evaluation tests for chemical substances). Although the normal intake quantity of AHCC is 1g per day, a megadose of 600g was administered during tests conducted on rats and no toxic effects were observed.

CONCOMITANT USE OF AHCC WITH ANTICANCER DRUGS

What kind of information is available regarding concomitant use of AHCC and chemotherapy drugs?

Prevention of side effects, tumor shrinkage, and prolongation of survival time have all been observed in animal tests on the concomitant use of cyclophosphamide (CY), bleomycin, 5-fluorouracil (5-FU), actinomycin D, mitomycin C (MMC), and adriamycin (ADr). It is believed that use of AHCC with most anticancer drugs will lead to life extension and prevention or reduction of side effects caused by anticancer drugs.

There are many reports regarding the efficacy of AHCC in reducing side effects caused by chemotherapy. In many cases, side effects like hair loss, bone marrow suppression (myelosuppression), loss of appetite, nausea, and vomiting have a profound effect on the quality of life (QOL), sometimes leading to termination of treatment. Animal test results have shown that AHCC can prevent the drop in immunity caused by chemotherapy.

So patients should avoid concomitant use of AHCC with immunosuppressants, such as those given at the time of organ transplantation.

Liquid diet and drugs are administered through the nose in patients at advanced stages of cancer. Can AHCC be taken together with these?

Administration of liquid diet through the nose is almost the same as oral intake. AHCC can also be taken through the nose by mixing it with the liquid diet formula. This, of course, requires the understanding and cooperation of the treating physician.

Are there any other effects of AHCC other than on the immune system?

Research results have shown that there are other effects of AHCC besides those on the immune system. Very simply, it normalizes the stomach condition and stimulates or improves appetite. There are also reports that it eases cancer pain and leads the patient toward mental and psychological stability. AHCC conditions the body as a whole and improves overall functioning.

Is AHCC safe for people with diabetes, chronic hepatitis (including types B and C viral hepatitis), high blood pressure, hyperlipidemia, rheumatism, asthma, and other chronic conditions?

It has been experimentally demonstrated that AHCC has therapeutic properties for diabetes, chronic hepatitis, high blood pressure, and hyperlipidemia. It is also believed that AHCC balances the immune system by suppressing the excessive "humoral" immune activity (Th2) that causes allergic disorders like rheumatism and asthma. There are reports of improvement in many of these disease conditions. However, in any of these disorders the original treatment must not be neglected and suitable advice from the doctor is strongly recommended.

Does immunity (that is, cell-mediated immunity) always improve as a result of taking AHCC?

The results of the tests conducted to study the cytokine-producing capacity of the immune system in patients and test animals taking AHCC have confirmed an increase in immunity in most cases. However, this is not always so. There are some cases where there is almost no reaction, depending on the constitution or condition of the person or animal taking the AHCC. It is necessary to think about using AHCC with other health foods in these cases.

What kinds of cancers is AHCC used to treat?

The reports available until now have been for the following cancers: brain tumors (primary brain tumor and metastatic brain tumor), cervical and cephalic cancers (tongue cancer, mesopharynx, and hypopharynx cancers), thyroid cancer, lung cancer, esophageal cancer, stomach cancer, carcinoma of the colon and rectum, liver cancer, gallbladder cancer, biliary tract cancer, pancreatic cancer, breast cancer, ovarian cancer, uterine cancer (cervical cancer and cancer of the uterine body), bone cancer, leukemia (acute leukemia, chronic myelogenous leukemia), multiple myeloma, and malignant lymphoma (Hodgkin's disease). Among these, there have been a large number of reports of treatment of liver cancer, breast cancer, lung cancer, and uterine cancer. Unfortunately, there have not been many cases in which AHCC has been concomitantly used with other medical treatments and which can be statistically analyzed. There is very little data on the sole use of AHCC for cancer. The Primary Surgery Group of the Kansai Medical University has concluded from the results of follow-up studies carried out over long periods that there has been a life-extension effect in hepatocellular carcinoma patients.

Can patients take AHCC to prevent recurrence and metastasis after surgery?

There are cases of using AHCC with anticancer drugs as well as using it alone to prevent postsurgical recurrence and metastasis. The preventive effect of AHCC against postsurgical recurrence of liver cell carcinoma has been confirmed scientifically, and prevention of liver cancer and skin cancer has been confirmed experimentally.

Are there any health foods that have stronger effects than AHCC?

There are very few health foods that have undergone the level of research that has been performed on AHCC, which makes comparison among other health foods difficult, especially when it comes to their relative efficacy in addressing issues relating to cancer. Although AHCC cannot easily be compared with other health foods, from the standpoint of its therapeutic effects, its reliability has been proved conclusively from this body of research and its widespread use in clinical trials.

What dosage of AHCC should be given to animals?

The standard doses are:

- Large dogs: 2–3g per day
- Medium-sized dogs: 1–2g per day
- Small dogs: 0.5–1g per day
- Cats: 0.5–1g per day

Conclusion

The future looks bright for AHCC because research carried out in Japan, China, the United States, and Thailand shows that it works both for prevention and treatment of numerous diseases for which conventional medicine has inadequate countermeasures. AHCC improves the immune system's ability to recognize tumors; it strengthens the effects of chemotherapy, protects the immune system from chemotherapy side effects, and prevents metastasis; it protects the liver; it guards against viral infections; and as of publication of this book there is research under way to test the protective properties of AHCC from the H1N1 (swine flu) virus at South China Agricultural University.

AHCC is anti-inflammatory, which is measurable by its effect in reducing a substance called CRP (C-reactive protein). C-reactive protein is high when there are infections, inflammatory bowel disease, hepatitis, pancreatitis, and some cancers. Inflammation drives the progression of cancer. Inflammation also plays an important role in cardiovascular disease. In cardiovascular disease, there is a strong relationship between circulating CRP, heart attacks, and strokes. AHCC has demonstrated its ability to reduce inflammation, and the resulting high levels of CRP. It is possible that the anti-inflammatory properties of AHCC can prevent many diseases caused by an unresolved inflammatory process.

AHCC has been tested for safety in human studies in the United States at Yale University and it has been shown repeatedly to be safe with cancer chemotherapy, most recently in the United States at M.D. Anderson Cancer Center in Texas. Future research will no doubt uncover more applications for this safe and effective immune system supplement.

Glossary

Acetylate: Introduce an acetyl group into a molecule. The acetyl group is a component of many organic compounds, including acetic acid (vinegar), aspirin, and the neurotransmitter acetylcholine.

Active oxygen: Humans breathe in air and absorb oxygen into the body. This oxygen is used for the metabolism of food inside the body to generate energy. However, when energy is produced by means of this metabolism, part of the oxygen is transformed into active oxygen and causes oxidative stress in the body (aging, like "rusting"). Active oxygen is neutralized by natural antioxidant systems in the body. Oxidative stress is caused by environmental toxins (pesticides, chemicals) emotional stress, and numerous diet and lifestyle factors.

Adenoma: A benign tumor of glandular origin.

Adjuvant: A pharmacological or immunological agent that modifies the effects of other agents, drugs, or compounds.

Antibody: A protein used by the immune system to identify foreign objects, such as bacteria and viruses. Each antibody binds to a target called an antigen.

Apoptosis: Programmed cell death. It is part of the normal life cycle of the cell. It is different from necrosis, which is cell death caused by trauma to the cells. Some cancer cells avoid apoptosis, so inducing apoptosis in cancer cells causes them to die instead of surviving an excessively long time and continuing to reproduce. The process of promoting the apoptosis of cancer cells and suppressing the apoptosis of healthy cells is currently being researched.

Cell-mediated immunity: Also known as Th1 immunity, this is an immune response that does not use antibodies, but activates T lymphocytes, such as NK cells and macrophages, that destroy microbes, damaged or infected cells, and other antigens.

Corticosterone: A steroid hormone, secreted by the adrenal glands, with mild anti-inflammatory properties.

Cytokine: A chemical messenger secreted by immune cells that signal the type of response to antigens by the immune system. These immunomodulators include the interferons, the interleukins, tumor necrosis factor, and others.

Dexamethasone: One of the adrenal cortical hormones (steroids). Besides acting as an immunosuppressant, dexamethasone also destroys, with active oxygen, the organs that are vital for immunity, such as the thymus.

FNT: Abbreviation for ferric nitrilotriacetate. This chemical is known to generate active oxygen inside the body and damage various organs. It is used experimentally to induce oxidative stress.

Histological: Related to the tissues. Histology is the study of the body's tissues.

Humoral immunity: Also referred to as Th2 immunity, this immune response uses antibodies produced in the B-lymphocytes to identify antigens that trigger an immune response.

Immunomodulator: A substance that either suppresses or stimulates some aspect of immune system activity.

Interleukins: A group of cytokines that are primarily produced by and act on leukocytes (white blood cells) to signal the type of action required by the immune system.

Macrophages: White blood cells that engulf and digest cellular debris and disease-causing microbes.

Monosaccharides: Monosaccharides, also called simple sugars, are the most basic form of carbohydrate. Glucose, dextrose, and fructose are all monosaccharides.

Myelosuppression: Suppression of the bone marrow function. The bone marrow produces red blood cells, white blood cells, and platelets, so myelosuppression can result in anemia as well as impaired immunity.

Opportunistic infections: Infections that take hold when the immune system is weakened. MRSA (Methicillin-resistant *Staphylococcus aureus*) and *Candida albicans* are examples of microbes that cause opportunistic infections.

Oxidation: The combination of a substance with oxygen. Combustion is a common example of oxidation. In living systems, oxidative stress is caused by an imbalance between the production of reactive oxygen and a biological system's ability to readily detoxify or repair damage from the resulting free radicals, the intermediaries of the reaction.

Polysaccharides: Complex carbohydrates, including starches, cellulose, and in the body, glycogen, which is stored in the liver and broken down into the monosaccharide glucose (blood sugar) and released into the blood when necessary.

Psycho-oncology: A new field of study, developed within oncology, which studies the effect of emotions on the immune system and the endocrine system, and the relationship between the emotions and cancer risk.

SOD: Abbreviation for *superoxide dismutase*. This is a detoxifying enzyme in the body's natural antioxidant defense system, which removes the excessive active oxygen from the body and neutralizes the effects of oxidative stress.

Viral load: A way to measure the severity of a viral infection by counting the amount of virus in the blood or other body fluid.

Suggestions for Further Reading

Books

Boik, John. *Natural Compounds in Cancer Therapy: Promising Nontoxic Antitumor Agents from Plants and Other Natural Sources.* Princeton, Minn.: Oregon Medical Press, 2001.

Cheung, Peter C. K. *Mushrooms as Functional Foods.* Hoboken, N.J.: John Wiley & Sons, 2008.

Kenner, Dan. *The Whole-Body Workbook for Cancer.* Oakland, Calif.: New Harbinger, 2009.

Pescatore, Fred. *The Allergy and Asthma Cure.* New York: John Wiley & Sons, 2003.

Sompayrac, Lauren. *How the Immune System Works.* Malden, Mass.: Blackwell, 2008.

Stamens, Paul. *Mycelium Running: How Mushrooms Can Help Save the World.* Berkeley, Calif.: Ten Speed Press, 2003.

Further Reading Online

Immune system primer: www.leavesoflife.org/media/ImmuneSystem.ppt

Effects of stress on immunity: www.apa.org/journals/releases/bul 1304601.pdf

Stress immunity and cancer: www.stressandimmunity.osu.edu/

Immunity and viral infection: www.csun.edu/~cmalone/pdf589/ch19.pdf

Boosting NK cell activity:

www.reuters.com/article/pressRelease/idUS206367+06-May-2009+PRN20090506 (Supplements)

www.humourfoundation.com.au/index.php?page=356 (Humor)

www.busywomensfitness.com/immunesystem.html (Exercise)

Index

About the Author

A traditionally trained physician who has chosen to practice integrative medicine, Fred Pescatore, MD, MPH, is medical director of the AHCC Research Association, headquartered in Rye, New York. He currently has a private practice called the Centers for Integrative and Complementary Medicine with offices in New York City and Dallas. There he treats patients with diabetes, heart disease, hepatitis, and cancer, as well as those with more ordinary complaints, by employing a combination of both alternative and traditional Western medicine.

Dr. Pescatore's medical knowledge is based on his training at St. Vincent's Hospital, Mt. Sinai Medical Center, and St. Luke's/Roosevelt Hospital Center, all in New York City. Before beginning his own practice, Dr. Pescatore was associate medical director at the Atkins Center, the world's preeminent institution for complementary medicine. He received his master's degree in public health from Columbia University's School of Public Health and his medical degree from American University of the Caribbean School of Medicine.

Dr. Pescatore is the cohost of *Healthy by Nature*, a radio show that educates listeners on the use of nutritional supplements. It can be heard around the country on www.healthybynatureshow.com. He is the author of *The Allergy and Asthma Cure*, *Thin for Good*, and *Feed Your Kids Well* (this last volume was the top-selling children's health book of 2000). Dr. Pescatore is a frequent guest on major television newsmagazine shows.

Dr. Pescatore thinks that AHCC is the best dietary supplement to strengthen the immune system. As a doctor prescribing natural remedies in the clinic, he encountered various diseases (ranging from colds to cancer) caused by weakened immunity. He found that a patient who has a strong immune system can lead a long and healthy life.

Dr. Pescatore says, "I have been using AHCC for almost ten years. The first case in which I used AHCC was a case of hepatitis C. There is a high incidence of hepatitis C in the United States— almost an epidemic. It is a potentially fatal disease that has a silent progression. This patient was given 1g of AHCC three times a day and the viral load dropped 85 percent. This was a surprising result in a potentially fatal disease like hepatitis C and using AHCC we have been able to save a lot of lives. These days almost all my patients use AHCC. It has been proved that AHCC is very effective for colds and influenza. Patients who are taking 1g/day of AHCC are not affected by the common cold or influenza, even in the season when they are widespread.

"AHCC is also recommended for cancer patients. AHCC can support patients in many ways: It can increase the number of white blood cells, prevent or decrease hair loss, and improve overall mood, which is very important during the course of cancer treatment. I feel that AHCC is clinically useful for almost all patients. Until now I have used AHCC for the prevention of diseases like cancer, diabetes, heart disease, hepatitis, arthritis, the common cold, or influenza. However, I think that AHCC is effective not only for these diseases but also for other diseases in which the immune system is weakened. AHCC, which improves all conditions, can be taken by all of us whether we are affected by a disease or not. Treatment and prevention of disease are equally important. I think that AHCC plays a very important role in both of these aspects of health care."

Printed in the USA
CPSIA information can be obtained
at www.ICGtesting.com
CBHW071232230924
14796CB00008B/396